THE
THRIVING
PHYSICIAN

How to Avoid Burnout by
Choosing Resilience Throughout
Your Medical Career

GARY R. SIMONDS, MD, MHCDS | WAYNE M. SOTILE, PhD

Published by:
Studer Group
350 West Cedar Street, Suite 300
Pensacola, FL 32502
Phone: 866-354-3473
Fax: 850-332-5117
www.studergroup.com

ISBN: 978-1-62218-101-8

Library of Congress Control Number: 2018952411

The stories in this book are true. However, some names and identifying details have been changed to protect the privacy of all concerned.

Printed in the United States of America

To all the families of physicians out there. You selflessly share your loved ones and bear the heavy lifting of tending to their wounds. To Cindy, who exemplifies this notion. And to you, Wayne, who has proven that a man can have a mentor, and develop new best of friends, well into his later years.

—Gary Simonds, MD, MHCDS

To the thousands of physicians and medical families and the hundreds of medical organizations I have worked with over the past forty years. I admire your courage, commitment to excellence, and heroism. And to Mary, Rebecca, Greg, Macy, Wyatt, Julia, Mike, Ava, and Michael—you polish my soul.

—Wayne Sotile, PhD

Table of Contents

How This Book Came to Be (and Where We Hope to Go From Here)

This book arose out of a unique partnership between an academic neurosurgeon, Dr. Gary Simonds, and a clinical psychologist/organizational consultant, Dr. Wayne Sotile. Not only are we coauthors of *The Thriving Physician*, we've witnessed together, firsthand, how stress manifests in physicians' lives…and we've seen which tactics work and which don't. We hope the synergy created by our partnership serves the book well.

(Now, we trust you'll forgive us as we break into third-person voice for just a moment. Such linguistic awkwardness has long been the plight of the collaborative writer!)

Dr. Sotile is an authority on promoting physician and organizational wellness. He has developed great expertise in the field from treating and studying over fourteen thousand physicians in all stages of their careers. His experiences and research have focused on learning both from those physicians and medical families who have thrived and those who have experienced significant difficulty handling the medical experience (i.e., gotten into trouble personally and/or professionally due to maladaptive behaviors).

Dr. Simonds is a seasoned neurosurgeon who runs a neurosurgery department and residency training program. His commitment to instilling a healthier way of approaching life "in the trenches" for all his team members led to his partnering with Dr. Sotile. Dr. Simonds challenged Dr. Sotile to engage a group of providers whom Dr. Simonds felt were on the far end of the bell-shaped curve for daily exposure to medical, psychological, and moral stressors and challenges: the members of his neurosurgery department.

Dr. Sotile's interest was piqued. Neurosurgery was the mysterious "Dark Continent" of medicine that few ventured near, and even fewer understood. As with Jane Goodall and her chimpanzees, Dr. Sotile embedded himself within the neurosurgery team, garnering trust, confidence, and fellowship. The team soon opened up and shared their experiences, allowing the two of us to study the "stress cauldron" that is neurosurgery.

We met with the entire neurosurgery team monthly over several years. We surveyed the team extensively, looking for indications of burnout potential, depression, anxiety, frustration, compassion fatigue, and anger, as well as for resiliency tendencies and skills.

Over time, we developed a program to help ameliorate the stressors and build resilience. We employed multiple strategies (many of them novel) to help team members weather, and even prosper, from the emotional, psychological, and physical challenges of the specialty. We found that relatively basic and straightforward interventions (through guided evaluation, discourse, and education) could have a profoundly positive impact on coping skills and behaviors. The effort is now in its fifth year.

Our Hope for You

Our program continues with new discoveries and insights encountered in every session. So much was gained in this experience that we felt that it should be shared with others. That means **YOU**! Our hope is that the discussions and recommendations of this book will help you to prosper psychologically as you face your own myriad of challenges.

First, one caveat: No matter how inherently hardy or well-trained in resilience tactics and strategies you may be, your ultimate well-being will hinge on a combination of individual *and* organizational factors. Physician well-being is directly affected by factors such as levels of workload, demand, decision latitude, autonomy, flexibility, support, and control in the workplace.[1] Fostering a **positive work environment** is therefore critical to any effort to build and perpetuate resilience. You cannot therefore be passive about your work environment. If it is lacking, you must seek to be a change agent for the positive.

Consider the many things that creative organizations are now doing to move beyond the "blame the victim" mentality that sometimes underpins physician resilience training (i.e., "learn to take a deep breath, then stop whining and get back into the chaos that is your workplace!").

Examples of What Other Creative Organizations Are Doing to Optimize Physician Support and Curb Physician Burnout:

Tactic	Organization
Administrators and support staff leaders round on physicians to solicit input and offer support	University of Alabama at Birmingham Health System, Birmingham, AL
Regularly survey physicians and other clinicians, and provide special consultation to those "high opportunity" work units that show elevations in assessments of burnout and/or sub-par levels of satisfaction and engagement	Mayo Clinic, Rochester, MN
Provide a team to assist with documentation	Cleveland Clinic, Strongsville, OH
Facilitate prescription renewals	Allina Health Cambridge Clinic, Cambridge, MN
Allow for documentation time mid-day	Northeast Georgia Physicians Group, Gainesville, GA
Provide staff help with physician e-mail inbox management	Fairview Clinic, Minneapolis, MN

Regularly offer specialized physician development programs such as Women in Medicine and Medical Families Today	Centura Health Penrose-St. Francis Medical Center, Colorado Springs, CO Ohio State University Wexner Medical Center, Columbus, OH Oregon Medical Group, Eugene, OR Carilion Clinic, Roanoke, VA Atrium Health, Charlotte, NC
Provide physician leadership development	FirstHealth of the Carolinas, Pinehurst, NC Carilion Clinic, Roanoke, VA CoxHealth, Springfield, MO Atrium Health, Charlotte, NC
Implement work flow redesigns to improve practice efficiencies	Avera Health, Sioux Falls, SD Medical Associates Clinic and Health Plans, Dubuque, IA ThedaCare, Oshkosh, WI
Develop offices for coordinating and delivering a wide range of physician support services	Adventist Florida Hospital, Orlando, FL Ochsner Health System, New Orleans, LA Loma Linda University Health, Loma Linda, CA Hennepin County Medical Center, Minneapolis, MN
Develop physician preference cards to facilitate cross-disciplinary collaboration	HSHS Sacred Heart Hospital, Eau Claire, WI
Provide physician support groups	Methodist Healthcare, San Antonio, TX Mayo Clinic, Rochester, MN

Regularly facilitate administrator/physician dialogues regarding physician needs and opinions	Mayo Clinic, Rochester, MN Vancouver Clinic, Vancouver, WA Centura Health Penrose-St. Francis Medical Center, Colorado Springs, CO Mission Health, Asheville, NC
Utilize LEAN principles to improve workflow efficiencies	Denver Health, Denver, CO Michigan Medicine, Ann Arbor, MI
Facilitate flexible and creative work/life integration strategies such as providing valet services and allowing physicians options about how and when they work (with fair adjustment in commensurate compensation)	Vanderbilt University School of Medicine, Nashville, TN Stanford University School of Medicine, Stanford, CA Mayo Clinic, Rochester, MN
Share cost savings with physicians	Atrium Physicians Network, Charlotte, NC
Share care among team members	Clinica Family Health, Denver, CO Department of Family Medicine, University of Colorado Health System, Denver, CO
Adjust RVU metrics to reflect the range of physicians' work	Ohio State University Wexner Medical Center, Columbus, OH
Offer physicians talent and career management coaching	Ohio State University Wexner Medical Center, Columbus, OH Carilion Clinic, Roanoke, VA Atrium Health, Charlotte, NC FirstHealth of the Carolinas, Pinehurst, NC

Provide resilience training	Virginia Tech Carilion School of Medicine and Research Institute, Roanoke, VA
Create opportunities for physician collegiality	Advocate Good Samaritan Hospital, Downers Grove, IL Mayo Clinic, Rochester, MN Centura Health Penrose-St. Francis Medical Center, Colorado Springs, CO

Sources: Personal consulting experiences [2-9]

We applaud these organizations for tackling this very real, very serious issue. Helping physicians cope with the immense stress they face is not only the right thing to do, it's a proactive move toward providing ever better patient care and organizational performance. We hope this book will play a role in sparking discussion across the industry—and ultimately will serve as an impetus for helping other healthcare organizations make needed changes that lead to improved physician well-being.

We realize fully that you, the individual physician, would effect many such changes if only you could. Physicians at all stages of the career journey lament their lack of control over the many factors that shape their work life. But we propose that you have more control than you might think. (More about this as we move along.)

> *Our coaching mantra and our resilience challenge is simple: "Even if 'they' are 90 percent of the problem, what's the 10 percent you are willing to own in order to foster your personal resilience?"*

We'll say up front that there are two things you can do to build resilience and prevent burnout. First, bring **positivity** to the workplace. When you do, you will engender it in return—often greatly magnified. Everyone expects you to be grumpy and bedraggled. Blow their minds by greeting your world with a smile and an engaged and appreciative attitude. Second, **take care of yourself and nourish the relationships that are important to you.**

If you can successfully do these two things throughout training and your medical career, you don't need this book! It's written for the vast majority of physicians who find them difficult due to the "slings and arrows" and distractions of a busy medical career. We will make you aware of the many challenges that make these vital activities more difficult, and we will show you many strategies to re-implant them into your persona and your day-to-day existence. We are so happy that you are joining us for this ride!

INTRODUCTION

It's a Doctor's Life for Me!

Ten years ago
I turned my face for a moment,
and that became my life

—*David Whyte,* The Heart Aroused

Macbeth: Cure her of that! Canst thou not minister to a mind diseased, pluck from the memory a rooted sorrow, raze out the written troubles of the brain, and with some sweet oblivious antidote cleanse the stuffed bosom of that perilous stuff which weighs upon her heart.

Doctor: Therein the patient must minister to himself.

—*William Shakespeare,* Macbeth

Becoming a physician is difficult. Life as a busy practicing physician is even more difficult. Yet, some hearty congratulations are in order. You made it! You are among an elite group; you fulfilled your dreams and are soon to be, or already are, a bona fide doctor! The challenge is enjoying the journey—and that's why we wrote this book.

This is not the typical handbook that teaches you how to manage hospital services, to multitask, to organize your workday, or to make the right diagnostic and therapeutic decisions. Rather, it is **a survival guide for your psyche.** Our goal is to teach you invaluable skills for taking care of yourself and the relationships that sustain you and help you grow. We believe that, if you are to thrive as a physician, learning these skills is as important as learning those that allow you to deliver excellent patient care. You cannot do the latter without the former.

Luckily for you, "times are a-changing." The cost of the culture of self-sacrifice and self-denial that has forever characterized life in medicine is now being called into question.[1] The fall-out of rampant physician burnout and maladaptive responses to daily stressors—from medical school to residency and beyond—has seized national attention. Organizations such as the ACGME, the AMA, and numerous national specialty societies have clearly taken notice.

Increasingly, focus is turning to lessons from the flip-side of burnout and distress: **resilience**. Resilience is the process of getting through difficult times and emerging stronger. We know that resilience is not solely an individual matter. Medical organizations, medical families, and individual physicians must partner to foster sustainable resilience. We also now know that resilience is not a pre-set or inflexible trait; and we know that it's not about being strong or smart or self-confident. Rather, resilience comes from a set of life-management skills that can be learned, developed, and practiced over time.[2]

Resilience is a key survival tool that can be strengthened with attention and practice. It is a critical factor in maintaining your psychological wellness. Through our personal (G. Simonds) and clinical (W. Sotile) experiences over the past four decades, we have found that the more resilient a physician learns to be, the more likely he or she will lead a happy, fulfilling, and productive career.

This Stuff Can Be Learned! We Wrote This Book To Teach You About It!

We are driven by our dual concern for your well-being and that of your patients. Research shows that, if it goes unchecked, the psychological toll of medical training and practice can spawn an array of maladaptive coping behaviors that compromise your resilience, disrupt your ability to collaborate, and thwart your effectiveness in patient care. It can turn you into a narcissistic jerk! Too often, the strain inherent in practicing medicine drains its practitioners of two essentials for providing extraordinary patient care: empathy and compassion.

We hope to help you learn how to assess your coping reserves and refill your energies when needed. For those just beginning this journey, we hope to help you develop an array of resilience skills that will serve you, right from the outset. For practicing physicians, we urge you to believe that it's never too late to choose resilience.

To the many cynics out there: Our approach goes beyond "psychobabble." The strategies and tactics we recommend are the evidence-based "pearls" derived from the fields of resilience, positive psychology, human motivation, organizational development, leadership, family systems, and more. Renowned resilience researchers have shown that, even in the face of contextual demands that are unrelenting (e.g., military combat), resilience training for high performers can yield transformational results.[3]

Integrating resilience training into your training experience and/or your medical practice is a worthy endeavor. Ideally, it should be inculcated into your overall curriculum and/or your team function. At the very least, we urge you to incorporate resilience boosts into your own day-to-day medical experience. ***You are worth caring for!***

Why This Matters

Consider the journey that is a medical career. From day one, you are in the thick of it. You survive the herd-culling cattle call of undergraduate pre-med "education" and the torture of the MCATs. You make it into a reputable medical school. There you try to assimilate a million points of data and get your first taste of extreme self-denial, brutal hours, and sleep deprivation. You continue to achieve scholastically in the ever-more competitive race for a "choice" residency slot. Then comes the soul-crushing experience of said residency. Then, the unsteady days of your early career, followed by the hyper-productive, hyper-fatiguing world of mid-career. Finally, after the waning years of what's hopefully a successful career, you "hang up your cleats," settle down on some remote ranch in Montana, and write your memoirs.

You know now, or you soon will, that the going is tough. And all the money you may earn, and all the societal approbation you may receive, won't completely soften the blows. The practice of medicine takes its toll: on your relationships, your family, your free time, your hobbies, your body, your youth—but most of all, on your psyche. Post-traumatic stress, compassion fatigue, disillusionment, resentment, burnout, depression, relationship tensions, work/family conflicts—these and other psychosocial struggles are rife.

No matter how committed and dedicated you are to your career, you will be vulnerable to the struggles. In the privacy of our coaching, counseling, and mentoring sessions with residents and practicing physicians, we hear evidence of this concept, almost daily:

- "If I had known a career in medicine would be this grueling, I'm not sure I would have signed on."
- "I see senior residents filled with confidence, and I doubt that I'll ever get there. My doubt in my own abilities is only deepening."
- "I lowered my head and drove, expecting it to all be easier after getting out of residency. It only got harder."
- "When do I reach the finish line? I have been working like a dog for decades, and there's no end in sight."
- "My family has no notion of what this is like. They just keep saying, 'We believe in you.' I appreciate that. Problem is, I'm not sure what I need to do to survive this."
- "My relationship with my fiancé? What relationship? We have so little time together, things between us never get on, and stay on, a good track."
- "I woke up this morning and realized that I was old. Where did it all go? Why did I work so hard? What do I have to show for it?"
- "My family says I work too much; my colleagues say I'm not working enough."

In this book, we call attention to the psychological and psychosocial "underbelly" of life in medicine that is too often ignored. We offer evidence-based recommendations on how to stay resilient and well through your medical training and beyond, all the way to the end of your career. It is never too late to shift gears and start focusing on your own wellness.

For some of you, this book will shed a compassionate light retrospectively; the concepts we present will help you to make sense of what you experienced in the earlier stages of your career. Those of you who are just starting out in medicine will find this book to be a roadmap for identifying potential pitfalls and a source of positive coping solutions. Experienced physicians will find a plethora of practical strategies and tactics for deepening resilience, personally and in their families and teams.

Merely working in medicine puts you at substantial risk of emotional and psychological distress. Medicine is a high-end, high-stakes, rapidly changing, multi-tasked field that exposes you to poor outcomes, human tragedies, human depravity, risk of litigation, unrelenting demands, bone-wearing fatigue, relationship disruption, isolation, loneliness, self-doubt, and more. And this exposure takes its toll. No wonder nearly one in every two physicians experiences severe burnout, significant work/home conflict, or other maladaptive sequelae.[4,5]

Frighteningly but not surprisingly, evidence has mounted that from residency onward, as physician wellness suffers, so too does the quality of medical and surgical care.[6,7] Thus, your resilience to the stressors of a career in medicine affect your wellness, that of your family, and to no small degree, that of your patients.

The real onslaught begins during training, a crucible from which few escape completely unscathed. Some seem better suited for the experience, but **none are immune**. The interplay of the tremendous daily physical, intellectual, and emotional challenges with your unique personality and coping style determines your levels of functioning, fulfillment, and satisfaction or distress, throughout the experience. It also greatly affects your growth and development, both as a physician and as a person. Coping patterns learned during training may impact and permeate a physician's entire life—for better or worse. And, if exposed relentlessly to toxic stress, even the hardiest of people will lose their ability to cope.

Please Don't Stop Reading. We're Getting to the Good News!

Practicing medicine should be a most fulfilling experience, even amidst the stresses, changes, and challenges you are facing. As we will discuss extensively, resilience hinges on honing your ability to harvest "uplifts" while enduring the hassles. Doing so helps practicing physicians reap the joy inherent in helping others and quietly bask in the self-affirmation that comes with constantly expanding their professional and interpersonal competence and confidence.

Medical training, too, can and should also be a time of joy of learning. Most medical trainees report a deep pride of affiliation, and a sense of having entered an elite corps of like-minded champions who survived the gauntlet of pre-medical education, and are now getting to hone skills that few people in history have developed. As your training progresses, you will likely note deep satisfaction and quiet pride in your growing sense of competency. And once you're over the hump of the first couple of years of residency, you will likely notice an expanding view that the "light at the end of this tunnel" is actually within sight. We urge you to harvest and relish these good and affirming feelings during these years, because you will need them.

> *In one way or another, most early- and mid-career physicians we coach or counsel express the following sentiment: "If I had known during my medical training that it would end well, that I would, indeed, make it, I believe I would have enjoyed it more. My anxiety and fear of failing during those years blurred my vision of so many of the amazing and exciting parts of the experience—aspects that I have learned to relish, in retrospect."*

In order to slay a fearsome beast, we need to know more about it: where it lives, what it looks like, what it feeds on, and so forth. So before we talk about building resilience, let's learn a little more about who is susceptible to burnout and how it manifests.

Let's Talk About Burnout and Other Struggles Physicians Face

Burnout is a state of physical, emotional, and mental exhaustion. It results from intense involvement with other people in situations that are emotionally demanding over extended periods of time.[8] If these interactions are emotionally draining, they may "empty your tanks" to the point that coping with anything becomes near-impossible. Key elements of burnout include overall emotional exhaustion (particularly at, or gearing up for, the workplace); depersonalization (loss of empathy; going numb); a sense of inefficacy (accomplishing less); and cynicism (about what one is accomplishing or can accomplish).

Burnout is an old concept that is frighteningly applicable to life in medicine. Just consider the following oft-quoted list of "You might be at risk of burnout if…" statements:[9,10]

- You work exclusively with distressed persons.
- You work intensively with demanding people who feel entitled to assistance in solving their problem(s).
- You are charged with responsibility for too many people.
- You feel strongly motivated to work with people, but are prevented from doing so by too many administrative tasks.
- You have an inordinate need to save people from their undesirable situations but find the task impossible.
- You are very perfectionistic.

- You feel guilty about your own human needs.
- You are idealistic in your aims.
- You tend to champion underdogs.
- You are frustrated by variety, novelty, or diversion in your work life.
- You lack criteria for measuring "good-enough" success, but have a strong need to know you are doing a good job.

Sound familiar? If you are being honest, you likely checked at least a few items on this list. Most physicians agree that the list offers a chilling description of their professional lives.

Perhaps most often, burnout is signaled when the energy required to cope adaptively (in a way that results in what is desired) with your interpersonal demands of life becomes depleted, and your typical recovery strategies—a night of good sleep, or a day off, or a workout at the gym, or spending time with the family—no longer rejuvenate you. In other words, your tanks of emotional energy become emptied, and nothing you do refills them quickly enough. This, in turn, compromises your ability to deal with others.

Think of burnout as being the "antithesis of engagement"—with a twist. Burnout is not a malady of the lazy. Rather, it's the committed, devoted physician who is most at risk. The "twist" comes with context: Burnout seems to flourish when a dutiful, mission-focused person works in a chronically frustrating setting. Management flaws, dysfunctional or unrealistic work environments, and/or poor self-management can all contribute to the condition.

Your risk of burnout increases if…

- Your personal values and goals are at odds with those of your work environment.
- You have limited control over how you go about meeting expectations that are placed upon you in your workplace.
- You work in a setting where you are rarely shown appreciation, or are rarely rewarded by leaders or management.
- Interpersonal tensions and conflict abound in your workplace.

The slippery slope of burnout leaves you feeling disconnected, unmotivated, fatigued, non-contributory, and eventually jaded about your contribution to the effort at hand. Energy, dedication, and pride are degraded, and diminished accomplishment follows.

Burnout is not necessarily a chronic condition; it signals temporary depletion of coping reserves. Furthermore, Christina Maslach emphasizes that burnout is not a dichotomous phenomenon (i.e., you are either burned out or you are not burned out). Rather, burning out occurs along a continuum that progresses from engagement, to feeling ineffective and overextended, to disengagement, to burning out.[11]

Burnout should be taken seriously. Chronically ignoring burnout can lead to clinical depression, somatic ailments, and a host of maladaptive personal and work behaviors and outcomes. These include but are not limited to the following:[12]

Emotional Exhaustion: You feel emotionally drained from your work, and become increasingly more frustrated and irritated when reacting to routine demands from patients and colleagues. Routine time off from work no longer rejuvenates you.

Impaired Cognitive Functions: Memory, concentration, and attention start to lapse, especially during the later stages of a demanding workday. To compensate, you rigidly rely on overlearned ways of thinking and behaving.

Depersonalization: Your work seems to have hardened you emotionally or made you more callous toward others. It's as though you are losing compassion for patients and colleagues.

Diminished Sense of Personal Accomplishment: Questions about whether your work really makes a difference haunt you, and you lose passion and motivation for work.

Impaired Performance: Work-related mistakes increase in frequency.

Physical Wearing-Down: Your body starts to show signs of wear and tear as your stress-related physical symptoms increase.

Emotional Distress Dispersion: Increasingly, you take work-related frustration home. Your irritability, worry, or anger at the end of a workday contaminates your home life. Soon, both home and work are affected by your overt or covert expressions of resentment. You feel misunderstood in both arenas.

Organizational Distress: As your negative moods affect those around you, incidences of complaints regarding inappropriate workplace behaviors rise, staff morale dips, and recruitment and retention of key employees becomes difficult.

The concept of professional burnout has garnered widespread popular attention in many fields, but particularly in medicine. Burnout, however, is only one of the many maladaptive responses to the stressors of a medical career. Psychological distress, depression, over-indulgence, divorce, loss of social networks, substantial decrement in performance, disenfranchisement, and more plague many in the field. We seek to arm physicians with a "toolbox" of methods to help prevent and ameliorate the impact of not only burnout, but of the many other sometimes devastating psychological ill-effects of a career in medicine.

We propose that every physician should work on his or her ability to weather the unavoidable stressors of the field and come through them psychologically stronger than before. This is the bedrock of the concept of "resilience"—*that is, to get through difficult times or experiences and grow from them.*

In short, we wish to help build resilient physicians—ones who engage in self-compassion and self-care throughout their careers. We assert that you, as a resilient physician, will avoid many of the psychological potholes that so many of your colleagues fall into, and know how to ride over them without becoming completely derailed in your career and your life.

Building Resilience

Acknowledging the experiences that cause you stress is an important step in building resilience. Many of the stressors you encounter are beyond your control. But remember, even if you "own" only 10 percent of the problem (or its control), you have something that can be positively addressed and perhaps affected.

Reminding ourselves of this helps counter the demoralizing self-criticism that all of us in medicine seem so prone to. It allows us to approach problems with a more resilience-boosting inner and interpersonal dialogue. Something like this: "These challenges are a tough part of medicine; they would be stressful for anyone. Everyone has a choice in deciding how to cope with stuff like this. How might I best manage my reactions to them?"

When you reflect on your stressors or discuss them with others, consider these key concepts:

- Go for supportive (not judgmental or dismissive) responses from trusted others (including yourself!).
- Deploy "reframing" strategies that move you to broader frames of reference (broader perspectives) with respect to your stressors.
- Try to learn different ways to face the inevitable coping challenges of your experience. (The stressors are not going to go away.)
- Note that self-compassion does not make you weak, whiny, or complacent. Research has shown that self-compassionate people are more resilient, less brooding, and more interpersonally effective.[13]

Self-Compassion

The remainder of this book is filled with strategies and tactics for curbing burnout by building resilience. But first, we'd like to mention a mindset we hope you will deploy as you move forward: *self-compassion*. This is a critical ingredient to fortifying yourself against the daily assaults upon your happiness, self-worth, sense of security, worldview, empathy, and psyche.

Self-compassion is not the same as self-pity, selfishness, or self-indulgence. It means granting yourself permission to take care of yourself as generously as you take care of others. In fact, it means making this self-care routine. Surviving a career in medicine is not unlike having to perform as an elite athlete year after year. Along the way, you encounter an array of bumps, bruises, and outright injuries—some physical, most psychological. To stay healthy, you will have to learn to prevent injury as much as possible and tend to those injuries that do occur.

Self-compassion is not easy in a profession that demands self-sacrifice and self-denial, and affords little time for reflection. In fact, the prolonged exposure to unrelenting stress you experience compromises (more like "beats down") the very capacity required for effective self-compassion. Acts of self-compassion won't come to you spontaneously. You will need to mindfully devote energy to them, energy that at times will feel sorely lacking.

Probing Questions and Quotes

Throughout this book we will provide many quotations and pose discussion questions to you (a few in each chapter and many more posted on our supplemental website). Please don't blow past them. The quotations should spur some interesting and deep thought (and hopefully a few smiles) related to the subject at hand.

The questions should greatly deepen and intensify the contemplation. Take on one or two at a time and don't rush through them. They will encourage some introspection and reflection—tools important in fortifying your emotional intelligence and establishing a solid routine of self-compassion. We see the questions as critical fuel for your resilience-building.

If possible, discuss some of the questions, along with your related observations and discoveries, with peers, friends, families, mentors, or perhaps a therapist. Personal growth is aided by at least some degree of social discourse and social support. Some find group discussions with colleagues helpful; others prefer doing so with a trusted friend, colleague, or loved one. Do what feels best for you. Compassion, affirmation, and empathy from others—in any form—helps to open us to positive internal changes, especially changes involving learning to better care for ourselves.

If you are tackling this on your own, be self-supportive and beware of self-criticism. We in medicine are a highly self-critical lot. It is part of our training. Counter this by working to develop a supportive and compassionate "alter ego"—a more nurturing and affirming aspect of yourself that can help you stay the resilience course. In other words, cut yourself some slack!

Enumerating the Stressors

Shortly, we will review a long list of the stressors physicians routinely face. In addition to increasing your self-compassion and (hopefully) enlightening your support system, we start here for a strategic reason: "Going to the balcony" and looking compassionately yet honestly at yourself as you cope with various contexts of your personal and work life serves as the conceptual bedrock of counseling, psychotherapy, and cognitive/behavioral therapy.

Self-monitoring and/or self-evaluating can disrupt maladaptive coping patterns and promote more adaptive coping. Simply asking a question about a difficult issue directs one's "mental map" to thoughtfully attend to that issue. This is called the principle of "simultaneity": *Change about an issue begins to occur simultaneously with raising questions about it.* By acknowledging a difficult issue rather than avoiding it or allowing yourself to be numb to it, your mind automatically sets out to address it. You begin working on the problem as you are exploring it. As you engage in this process, you may encounter some surprises.

> *We asked CC-VTC residents to tally the number of unpleasant interpersonal interactions they encountered with coworkers per week. The residents reported totals in the 50 to 90/week range! And these rates were likely underreported!!*

In our sessions with physicians throughout the country, most routinely discover that not all stressors are externally imposed. Intrinsic characteristics and self-demands tend to create stressors as powerful as those experienced externally. For example:

> *In reviewing personality inventories taken by our team, we found that the majority had significant perfectionist tendencies. While a degree of perfectionism is certainly required in medicine, strong perfectionist tendencies can lead to a constant sense of defeat and frustration, particularly in a field of such challenging outcomes.*

Discussing your observations with others helps you realize that you are not alone and that your feelings and responses are not unique, or atypical, or silly, or weird. Thus, it is useful to tackle these subjects with colleagues. Bear in mind that, because attitudes and emotions are contagious in groups, "cataloging stressors" can devolve into aimless, unproductive complaining ("bitch sessions"). Likewise, cataloging only on your own may create a self-perpetuating loop or a sense of victimization.

So, make an effort to come up with positive and productive potential responses to these stressors as you think about them. The ultimate goal is to create supportive self-reflection and dialogue that helps you to problem-solve rather than just react or kick into maladaptive coping mechanisms (anger, resentment, isolation, etc.).

Share This Book!

We previously wrote a similar book, *Building Resilience in Neurosurgical Residents: A Primer*. Since its release, many readers noted how loved ones, family members, and friends would on occasion pick it up and leaf through it. They would soon find themselves engrossed and would approach the neurosurgeons, sometimes with tears in their eyes, and say: "I had no idea what you were going through." Many neurosurgeons have told us that this has opened up invaluable dialogue between them and those with whom they are close.

Many of us compartmentalize our "in-the-trenches" experiences when we finally escape the confines of our work settings. We may not want to relive many of the painful moments of the day, or we feel the hospital gets enough of us day to day, or we may want to spare our loved ones the nastiness of real-world medicine, or we may simply want to keep the two worlds separated. But it's not healthy to throw up barriers to communication about huge portions of our lives.

We believe it is critical to your resilience to remain intimately engaged in the relationships that are important to you. So share this book with those who matter to you—loved ones, friends, family members, significant others. It will help them better understand your world. It will help them with their own resilience as they suffer many of your stressors alongside of you. We are not advocating trying to solicit pity here; rather we are trying to help you keep connected with those you care about. Sharing this book will open up avenues of communication.

Finally, feel free to share this book with your colleagues. Not just other physicians, but also with hospital administrators, practice administrators, organizational leaders, and anyone else who might benefit from its message. The more our industry's leaders fully grasp the stressors we face—and the resilience-building techniques that can help alleviate some of our suffering—the better off we (and of course our patients) will be.

Healthcare is in a state of rapid change. Physicians are along for the ride, desperately trying to hang on. We need every possible resilience tool at our disposal. If you find solutions that work for you, please share them. The future you change for the better might just be your own.

Understanding Your World and the Challenges of a Career in Medicine

Doctors inhabit a rather surreal world. It's a world that most outsiders (and many insiders) have no real appreciation for with regard to its pressure-cooker stressors and mind-numbing idiosyncrasies.

One of the principal goals of this book is to provide strategies to help you cope with the various stressors that affect you, your performance, and your well-being. But first you need to recognize them and acknowledge their existence. We invite you to survey your "playing field" (or battlefield as the case may be) to better understand the coping challenges you face. We will arm you with a quiver of strategies to help you cope with and even grow from these challenges.

In this book, we list many of the challenges and stressors that physicians face in their day-to-day travails. We have included short analyses, some related thought-provoking questions, and some potential coping strategies for each issue. We hope that each stressor section may serve as a jumping-off point for related discussions. Think about what stressors clearly affect you the most and keep an eye out for those that do affect you but have previously gone unrecognized.

We encourage you to peruse the list and engage in reflection, introspection, internal dialogue, and preferably open discussion of one or two of the issues at a time. "Normalize" the fact that discussing such issues and shaping resilience will make you a better physician. Discuss some of the concepts with trusted colleagues and those close to you. Be patient with those who are not directly sharing the experiences with you. Focus on how certain situations affect you and those around you rather than dwelling on the issues themselves. Seek to understand and appreciate your environment and how to grow within it.

When discussing with others, offer appropriate self-disclosure and life lessons from your own experience. Use appreciative questioning. Think about similar situations and how you responded to them, and how they made you feel. Explore the phenomenology surrounding a specific issue (e.g., why would phone calls from one ICU often end in acrimony, and those from another not?). Inquire as to how and when the targeted issue affects your experience. Explore "best practices" that you discover in these considerations and discussions for dealing with an issue, and what you see as future challenges regarding it.

Remember, you are not supposed to have all the answers. These issues are the "stuff" of the psychosocial underbelly of the overall physician experience. Resilience hinges on accurately identifying and appropriately expressing this "stuff" and choosing to adaptively manage oneself in response to it—even if the challenges being faced cannot be resolved or eliminated.

Most of the following issues are somewhat generic to all physicians and other healthcare providers. Some may be more commonly encountered during training, others in the thick of a flourishing medical practice. Some may be more intensely represented in your institution than others. Some may not play a major role in your experience. If not, noting these stressors may boost your compassion for colleagues who are facing them.

Our list is not exhaustive, and you will probably come up with many more (we had to stop someplace!). We are very interested in hearing from you about challenges and stressors brought out in your own discussions, and how you (and perhaps your group) manage to cope with these. Please contact us through garyrsimonds@gmail.com. Discussions of many of these stressors can be accessed through our podcast on iTunes under the title "Surviving Residency."

CHAPTER ONE

Spring Forward? Can't We *Fall* Back?

Time Compression—Time Starvation

"How did it get so late so soon? It's night before it's afternoon. December is here before it is June. My goodness how the time has flown. How did it get so late so soon?"

—Dr. Seuss

"Pleasure and action make the hours seem short."

—*William Shakespeare,* Othello

All physicians pour inconceivable hours into their training, practice, and maintenance of proficiency. Sixty to eighty-hour in-hospital/in-office work weeks are not uncommon even for attending physicians in mature practices. Recent research has shown that, compared to other U.S. workers, sevenfold as many physicians work 60+ hours per week (42 percent of physicians versus 6 percent of U.S. workers).[1] Trainees spend up to 80 hours a week in-hospital and countless others reading and studying. For the average American full-time worker, 80 hours a week is the equivalent of almost *two* full-time jobs (statistically, the average American worker puts in 47 hours a week).[2]

What is more, there is almost no down time during the workday. The typical physician multitasks almost every minute of his or her workday. There are few breaks, and breaks when they come tend to be used for making calls or catching up on email. Meals are almost always taken on the run if at all. When physicians have the luxury of completing a solitary task, said task generally requires intense and sustained focus.

Now, we concede that the typical resident work week has been foreshortened from those of the days "when the giants walked the halls," but this has not been shown to greatly relieve the degree of time compression experienced in training. Many contemporary residencies use every minute of the 80-hour week in training their charges.

Clearly, patient care and documentation are far more complex and time consuming than they once were. Furthermore, resident duties have become more concentrated during the foreshort-ened workweek, shifting learning activities (and often clinical and documentation activities) to home. All in all, contemporary medical residents dedicate approximately the same amount of time to their training as did their predecessors, with the same work/life balance fallout.

> *Residents interviewed across the country reported that their average amount of "free time" per night was no more than one hour, and that was taken at the expense of their already-compromised sleep schedule (which they reported to be, on average, 4-6 hours per night). Many residents report-ed essentially no time spent on hobbies or external interests. Time spent en-joying loved ones fared no better. Many residents felt hopelessly behind in managing the mechanics of life such as taking care of banking, doing the laundry, running errands, shopping for food, getting a haircut, etc. Most felt a constant "pressure of time" both at work and when out of the hospital. Most confirmed time as one of the most "precious commodities" in their worlds.*

For the physician out in practice, things aren't much better. Responsibilities change, but the hours often remain substantial. Greater demands in documentation and compliance have ex-tended the physician's day well past the clinical activities. Most surveys have noted that the institution of the electronic medical record has actually lengthened the physician's day rather than shortened it. Many practicing physicians continue documentation efforts and "call-backs" from home, well into the night.

Furthermore, learning doesn't stop at the end of residency. Most specialties are under constant change, development, and refinement, requiring hefty yearly CME commitments and periodic

Maintenance of Certification examinations. Thus, time must also be devoted to professional reading and study.

Living in a time crunch may have both an immediate impact on your stress levels and a cumulative, erosive effect on your overall quality of life. "Time starvation" becomes part of the lifestyle, repeated day to day, month to month, year to year—perhaps throughout a career! This is a syndrome that should not be underestimated. No matter how motivated you are and how much you love your work, if you go too long before restoring your energy reserves for working—by pursuing other life interests and pleasures—**you will burn out**!

It is not the absolute hours that you work that can be so toxic, but rather the hours of rejuvenation (and living!) that you are losing. Practicing physicians tell us that they look back and recognize that they were totally absent from whole components of "normal" life during their residencies and in the first stages of practice. Many tell us they still are. Countless "date nights," Super Bowl parties, gatherings with friends and family, plays, musical events, movies, babies' first steps, had all vanished into the past. Holidays and birthday celebrations have been shifted to different weeks or missed altogether. But these are precisely the activities that will rejuvenate you.

What is more, chronic fatigue inescapably compromises the quality of available time. How often have you slept through a date night or some outing that was supposed to be "recess" time?

> One of our colleagues reported that, when he was a resident, his children literally believed that the living room couch was cursed. Every time he or his fellow resident friends would sit upon the couch, they would immediately fall into a deep, unrousable sleep. The children made sure to steer clear of the couch at all times lest they fall under the same spell.

One caveat: Long hours dedicated to work does not automatically equal burnout. You are likely to remain resilient despite working hard, long hours if you find your work meaningful, enjoyable, and rewarding. However, this principle will surely "fall off the table" if no time is left for rejuvenating activities, and the mental and physical drain of long hours has sapped all of your potential positive coping capability.

Here are a few questions for you to contemplate and discuss with your peers, friends, families, mentors, or perhaps a therapist. Please see www.studergroup.com/thriving-physician for more questions.

Consider and Discuss

- Do you sometimes stay at work when you don't need to? Why?
- How would you ideally construct a "free-time" schedule to optimize your time away from work? What would you do with free time in the evenings if you had no television, computer, or video games?
- How can you help make the work environment more light and enjoyable for yourself and those around you?
- Would you be willing to compromise on compensation for more free time?
- What are the special events of life outside of work that you really should not miss or compromise on?

Building Resilience

Remember that burnout correlates less with time spent at work than it does with a lack of enjoyment/fulfillment derived from work. Rather than see your work as drudgery, remind yourself of what drew you into medicine. Try to appreciate new learnings, special cases, adrenaline rushes, associating with colleagues, getting to know your patients, the humanity and grace of the sick and injured, the moments of humor, moments of pathos, the deep plunge into humanity, and more.

- Try to work *efficiently*. For example, seek help in making the EMR as efficient for you as possible. Share your secrets with coworkers!
- Beware of inertia. Time can be lost just by a slow ramping-up of productive activities.
- In the same light, beware of time sumps in the workplace: surfing the internet, playing video games, watching videos, etc. These eat up your productive time and fill you with guilt. Use small breaks with such activities as rewards for bursts of productivity.
- Beware of the same energy-draining time sumps when you get home. A certain amount of "decompression" is likely good for you, but total immersion in such activities every free moment is not.

- Get started early. Studies have shown that most of us are at maximum productivity in the early hours of the day and are at our least in the late hours of the evening. Don't allow your workday to "phase shift" to later and later starts and finishes.
- Create a work schedule. Appoint time for various activities and hold yourself to the schedule. This encourages you to use your time efficiently and to "get out of the blocks" quickly. Recognize what is critical to be accomplished in a certain timeline and prioritize your activities.
- Recognize that there will be many a day that you simply cannot complete all your tasks. Some non-urgent, non-essential tasks need to be released. They will pop up again if they truly need attention.
- Don't get bogged down in non-urgent electronic communications. Although they always seem to require immediate attention and reply, most do not. Dedicate one or two times a day to address electronic communications. Attend to the messages that are of significance.
- Give priority to tasks that are time sensitive and important, followed by those that are important but less time sensitive. Get to the others only if you can.
- Try to live for the moment and not the end of the day. Cherish those moments in the exam room and hospital floors. Connecting and bonding with your patients and fellow caregivers is a life-affirming experience that few others get to enjoy. Here's an exercise that may help: At the end of each workday, recall three events that were special, terrifying, hilarious, surprising, touching, or heart-warming. Think of three personal interactions that were rewarding. You're reframing your mental map to recognize events that make the day interesting, exciting, and fun.
- At home, participate. Turn the TV off for a bit and engage in an activity that you truly enjoy: play the guitar, go for a walk, work out, read a novel, paint/draw—whatever "floats your boat."
- Try to put off the "fire-gazing." Fire-gazing may indeed be necessary and restorative but the earlier you start, the longer you will go; you will likely regret the time lost in the activity and find that it left you more drained than rejuvenated.
- Check out some of the many time management books and courses out there (often oriented to the business world). Try some of their suggestions. Also, check out some of our efficiency suggestions in the following "Multi-Tasking" Section.
- Seek out, and make full use of, when possible, physician efficiency resources at your institution such as scribes, medical assistants, physician assistants, and nurse practitioners.

CHAPTER TWO

Another Assignment? Gee, Thanks!

The Curse of Multi-Tasking

"Multi-tasking is a lie."

—*Gary Keller*

"Beware the barrenness of a busy life."

—*Socrates*

Modern medicine makes "multi-taskers" of us all. We all have days filled with multiple patient care needs, escalating productivity expectations, and relentless demands for our time and attention. With the advent of the electronic medical record, we now spend a sizable portion of each day entering data and filling out mandatory "fields" within EMR programs. What's more, electronic medical record systems enable providers, nurses, even patients to contact you with the expectation of a prompt (if not immediate) response. You may also be hyper-accessible, like it or not, via cell phone, e-mail, text, Facebook, Twitter, Instagram, and the like. And you're likely subject to multiple institutional meetings scheduled to the convenience of administrators, not physicians.

Cognitive scientists point out that true **multi-tasking is a myth**. Rather, the human brain addresses multiple concepts and demands in series—it just switches between them rapidly. We shift our focus and attention from one task to another (and back again) so quickly that we think we are handling multiple tasks at once. What we're really doing is compromising our ability to effectively handle each task. The more tasks that are engaged, the slower the processing, the greater the error rate, and the greater the associated stress, strain, and anxiety.[1,2]

Medicine can be a work flow nightmare. You are expected to function in a near perpetual state of "multi-tasking" while simultaneously facing circumstances that demand your exquisite focus on a singular task. This type of environment can prove to be a minefield. So watch your step!

> *One of our residents was recently "written up" for "uncooperative behavior" due to the fact that he did not respond to repeated calls placed by a floor nurse in want of a laxative order for a patient. The resident in question was enmeshed in an emergent and protracted operation (severely broken spine). It being the middle of the night, no other team member was immediately available to answer the pages. The task fell upon the circulator nurse, who became so exasperated by the volume of calls that she turned the alarm off on the cell phone.*

When the demands are coming in much faster than they can be handled, you will be in a state of demand overload that will significantly stress you and put you at risk for behavioral "snaps" and forays into sarcasm and other anti-social responses.

> *One of our medical colleagues recalls how, when on-call as a resident, he would record his mounting task list on a yellow legal notepad. The tasks would rapidly stack up and fill an entire page as he serially addressed one problem after another. Some nights the pages and calls would come in so rapidly that he could not even keep up with the call-backs. He would fill up the entire page with the numbers he had yet to get to. The stress of not being able to address each problem was rough enough, but it became unbearable when he could not even attend to the incoming calls as the numbers on the page mounted.*
>
> *The phenomenon continues today. I (G. Simonds) was on call the other night and received six separate calls from the wards and four separate calls from the Emergency Room while I was taking a call from an*

> *outside physician through our Transfer Center. Despite 34 years of on-call experience, this still resulted in a sense of distress and tightness in the chest.*

Here are a few questions for you to contemplate and discuss with your peers, friends, families, mentors, or perhaps a therapist. Please see www.studergroup.com/thriving-physician for more questions.

Consider and Discuss

- When does multi-tasking become impossible? Can you tell when you are reaching your limit?

- Where do you notice yourself multi-tasking out of habit, even when the context does not require you to do so? Does the behavior carry over to home?

- How do you respond when you see a colleague being bombarded with tasks? Do you dive in and help?

- If you fall behind in your task list, what is the worst that can happen?

- How often do you actually say "no" to a non-essential request? How does that make you feel?

Building Resilience

When faced with multiple tasks at once, try to prioritize them and work off of a list. Group your tasks by urgency and importance. If you are not sure what items to place at the top of the list, ask senior colleagues for guidance. Realize you may not always accomplish the entire list. Delegate the less important, less urgent issues as much as possible, but check up on them periodically. Attend when possible to less urgent tasks that are liable to become urgent later on.

- Regroup frequently in the day. Rework the list as needed. Certain problems may have risen to the top; others may have gone away.

- Finish tasks you have started before moving to the next. It is inefficient to keep retreading the same task.

- Think geographically. Try not to bounce from one end of the hospital to the other and back.

- When feasible, offer help to others. You will feel less guilty about accepting help when you really need it.
- Batch similar or co-located tasks when possible, but be careful not to make the batches to large or lengthy.

CHAPTER THREE

No Pain, No Gain!

The Work Demands of a Career in Medicine

"A dream doesn't become reality through magic; it takes sweat, determination, and hard work."

—*Colin Powell*

"Success is no accident. It is hard work, perseverance, learning, studying, sacrifice, and most of all, love of what you are doing or learning to do."

—*Pelé*

Let's not beat around the bush here: Medicine is work, hard work. Every step of the medical journey requires intense commitment and much physical and mental "elbow grease." Just because you may work long, hard hours, however, does not mean you are more prone to burnout or other psychological fallout. Rather, work in a rewarding, interesting, exciting, challenging, interactive environment filled with meaning, shared focus, and daily uplifts will assure your resilience.

This is what makes medicine so special. Within it, there is a self-sustaining and rejuvenating engine that provides professional rewards for you that few other professions can. After all, how many other professions are solely dedicated to making life-changing differences for those in great distress?

But it is hard work, very hard work, and every physician can reach periods in their career where the weight of the work can make them lose the forest for the trees. In this chapter, we hope to scatter some breadcrumbs that will help lead you through the forest and reclaim the sense of wonder and dedication that medicine can so readily inspire, despite the commitment and hours.

Most students entering medical school recognize that medicine involves long hours and heavy workloads. Few, however, fully comprehend the degree to which this is true. Each stage of a medical career involves an element of culture shock. The transition from college undergrad to medical student is intense. The sheer volume of material that must be assimilated is unlike anything previously encountered. Many, however, find medical school supremely enjoyable. They already worked like dogs as undergraduates. There is little that is conceptually difficult—after all, it isn't particle physics. Memorization of vast amounts of information is the greatest challenge. But it is memorization of the stuff that they had always wanted to know. Many liken it to learning a new language. Once one catches on, it settles into an enjoyable tour through the mysteries of life.

For residents, the stakes are taken up a notch. In addition to digesting volumes of even greater information, residents become involved in high-level, tertiary medical center patient care from sun up to sun down. Intricate decision making, countless interpersonal interactions, long stretches of time on one's feet, extensive record keeping, and constant multi-tasking are the norm. Tasks are routinely sustained for 12-hour days and 28-hour call-shifts—often pushing the boundaries of the mandated 80-hour work week.

> *One of our colleagues grew up in a medical family. He witnessed his father working long hours, running out for calls in the middle of the night, and working many a weekend. Yet, he had no concept of just how hard he would work in his residency and for the rest of his professional life—it had to be experienced to be understood. When he set foot into his teaching hospital for the first day of residency, he felt like he had stepped onto a "runaway train." Yet, he loved every minute and would never have exchanged his training, his profession, his specialty, or his life for anything else.*

If you are a resident, you are expected to be a "jack of all trades." In addition to learning your specialty, prepping for various rounds and "inquisitions," medical consultation and care, procedures, and documentation, you will become responsible for:

- Teaching rotating students
- Counseling angry and grieving families
- Engaging in diplomatic interactions with other (often conflicting) services
- Tracking down missing materials
- Interpreting and interfacing with new technologies for aging faculty (a big one at our place—although a great source of resident mirth at least!)
- Troubleshooting dysfunctional technologies
- Acting as de facto therapist to and mobilizing your patients (when the therapists fail to show up)
- Acting as de facto specialists (when they fail to show up)
- Acting as a de facto social worker when your service is having trouble getting a patient out of the hospital
- Transporting patients
- Performing IV access, spinal taps, line placement, and other small procedures
- Interpreting radiology reports (when no one else can)
- Pestering diagnostic physicians for various "reads" and opinions
- Chauffeuring visiting dignitaries
- And much, much more…even though your "routine" medical demands in and of themselves would be enough to fill the 12-hour working day.

As a resident, there is little time to catch your breath. Food is usually gobbled down on the run. The work simply does not pause for such "pedestrian" bodily needs.

> *In recent discussions with leaders of physician wellness initiatives from two hallowed medical schools—Johns Hopkins and the University of Rochester—residents independently identified the same top three desires for improving their lots. These were: access to healthy food, decent drinking water, and the occasional bathroom break.*

In addition, "nights off" for residents are often dedicated to studying the science behind their given specialties, preparing for procedures, or writing research papers. Yet, every day of your residency, you gain new skills, new acumen, new competencies, deeper understanding, greater capabilities, a greater sense of medical nuance, and a greater capability to help others and affect their lives forever.

Now, once fully trained, it all downshifts to a life of ease and Wednesday afternoons out on the links, correct? Well, not really. People get sick and injured at all times of the day and night. Few practicing physicians have to worry about job security—the work is always there—only now with a much greater degree of responsibility. Practicing physicians generally work longer hours than any other professionals, take night calls with some regularity, and must perpetually seek to stay up to date with their professional and specialty advances.

In other words, there is a lifetime of hard work. Those who don't anticipate this are in for a career and quality-of-life letdown. Realizing that hard work is part and parcel to a career in medicine is the first step in learning how to derive satisfaction and even joy from that work. And so many do. Few careers inspire such levels of willful devotion and "after-hours" commitment. Few professions see such high percentages of participants plying their trade well into their seventies and even eighties. It isn't the remuneration or social approbation that drives your career, but rather an abiding love for the work.

Here are a few questions for you to contemplate and discuss with your peers, friends, families, mentors, or perhaps a therapist. Please see www.studergroup.com/thriving-physician for more questions.

Consider and Discuss

- Which aspects of your work do you hope to leave behind at the next stage of your training or career? Which aspects do you actually think you will leave behind? Are you being realistic?

- Is hard work a prerequisite for being a superlative physician?

- How hard do you intend to work throughout your career? How will you establish this level of work? Will you make compromises to establish this? Would you accept a decrement in pay to ensure a manageable workload? How much?

- What work is most enjoyable? What is insufferable? What makes the difference?

- How many days off do you have each month? How many should you have? How many do you plan to take in the future?

- Are there ways to take "micro-vacations" during your workdays? How?

Building Resilience

We know what you are going through. It is rough. But there *is* some rhyme and reason to it all. You are part of a noble cause: giving aid to those who are suffering. The more you pour into it, the more competent you will become and the more you will be able to contribute. You are one of the privileged few who has the intelligence, industry, perseverance, and supporting infrastructure to practice medicine in a miraculous age—and to help your fellow man.

To you residents out there, the ordeal may feel like hazing. To you practicing physicians, it may feel like a breach of the contract you made with yourself about your future life. But it does serve a lofty purpose: It makes *you* a superlative modern doctor.

- Take some time to grant yourself a feeling of pride and a sense of calling. For those in your early career stages, peer around the trees and envision the wonderful practitioner you will become, all the people you will help, and the difference you already make to so many. For those in mid or late career, pause for a moment and savor the supreme level of competency you have achieved, and how patient after patient invests complete trust in you and are thankful for your efforts—and will be so for the rest of their lives.

- Allow yourself to feel good about what you are doing. Hard work doesn't necessarily correlate with burnout if you feel engaged, motivated, and fulfilled in your work. If you can go home happy and satisfied with what you have done, the game is half-won! And your home life will flourish in return.

- Remember that **meaning is the antidote to burnout**, and your profession is abundant with meaning. Take moments every day to remind yourself that you are helping those who are in trouble—those who may be experiencing the worst moments of their lives. Take pride in this; let it fill you. Savor the happy satisfied exhaustion your hard work can bring (like after a long-distance run, or an intense work-out at the gym).

- On a practical side, remember this mantra: "If you wait to leave work until everything is done, **YOU WILL NEVER LEAVE**." Your daily workload is filled with endless lists of tasks that can never be completely accomplished. Many physicians have never learned to prioritize their endless work demands. They spend hours every day spinning their wheels, doing tasks that will have little or no impact on patient care.

Furthermore, many inefficiently handle their work volume, even if they have prioritized it well. Some feel they must participate in a twisted "*suffering contest*" with their colleagues—forever demonstrating that they work longer hours and take fewer breaks than anyone else. The net effect is additional hours in the workplace or, worse yet, dragging hospital and/or outpatient tasks home to be tackled in what should be time for soothing, reconstitution, and rebuilding. Think: How often do you work on the electronic medical record from home?

One of the greatest weapons against your daily workload is the ability to prioritize and efficiently handle your work tasks. A savvy physician can visit dozens of patients, write notes, perform a handful of procedures, teach medical students, handle some emergent consultations, check on colleagues or trainees, and still leave work at a reasonable hour. This is a skill. It is not intuitive. It has to be taught and learned and practiced.

- Learn to prioritize caring for patients by acuity: Consider who are the sickest. Who are the most vulnerable or unstable? Remember the translation of "triage" is "to sort." This is critical to your efficiency and effectiveness as a physician.
- Order the day. For a surgeon, it might be: Sickest patients first, pre-ops second, discharges third, routine patients next, charting, calls, results review, other tasks (such as forms).
- Shorten notes to the important information: status, changes, working hypothesis (about what you think is going on with the patient), plan, alternatives, critical labs, and studies.
- Don't go beyond your expertise. Focus on what you have been called in to do for the patient. Enlist other specialists for problems that go well beyond your expertise.
- Delegate what you can. All too often we physicians see ourselves as "lone wolves" in our fights with disease, but there are small armies around us who will help if we ask.
- Focus on what the patient is seeing you for, what their chief complaint is. If they present to you a laundry list of problems, consider breaking up the list to separate visits. Key phrases like "Mr. Jones, what problem is the one that is affecting you most?" or "Ms. Jones, what is the main reason you came to see me today?" might hone the problem list and allow you to streamline your clinical decision-making and utilization of time in the exam room.
- Leave when you can. Don't wait around and look for more work to fall upon you, because it will!

- Review the methods of the most efficient physicians, advanced care practitioners, and residents around you. Share secrets.
- Consider consulting efficiency and/or process experts. Big medical institutions often have related teams on staff.
- Seek efficiency but keep the personal touch.
- Offer assistance to your colleagues when they are bogged-down. They will return the favor!

CHAPTER FOUR

You Want Me to Come See What?

The Tyranny of Call

"This would simply be the best job in the world…if it wasn't for call!"

—*Gary Simonds*

"Interruptions can be viewed as sources of irritation or opportunities for service, as moments lost or experience gained, as time wasted or horizons widened. They can annoy us or enrich us, get under our skin or give us a shot in the arm. Monopolize our minutes or spice our schedules, depending on our attitude toward them."

—*William Arthur Ward*

The psychology of the on-call experience is one of the most frequently underestimated "underbelly" aspects of life in medicine. Recent research shows the number of nights per month spent on call correlates linearly with physician levels of burnout and with physician marital dissatisfaction.[1,2]

Frequent call not only leads to sleep loss, but has an insidious impact on the psyche of a physician. Physicians and their families typically expect to sacrifice much of their personal life to work. Call, however, invades the physician's home and changes his or her very "presence" there.

Beware the "On-Call Syndrome"

You cannot master a coping challenge that remains unrecognized. So, let's first shine a light on the "on-call syndrome." We hear routinely from life mates of physicians that the typical physician on call is not the same animal that he or she is off of call. This includes you!

In addition to the obvious restrictions of being on call—you cannot drink alcohol or leave the geographic area—there is quite an abnormal psychology to the whole experience. During a night of call, you must be ready to leap into extremely serious and technically challenging situations immediately. As such, you are perpetually on alert—anticipating interruption.

If you are like many physicians, you may be superstitious about call and may avoid many enjoyable activities for fear of inciting the "pager gods." You may believe that if you think the wrong thoughts you will be punished. You may reach the point that you can't even look at your cell phone for fear you will set it off. If so, you are in good company—these are all common on-call sentiments experienced by your colleagues.

> At our institution, there are patients ("frequent fliers") who simply cannot be mentioned as call closes in—"One breath about 'John Smith' and he invariably shows up in the emergency room with a major problem." If that patient is mentioned, the poor sod who does so can anticipate withering stares and oaths of vengeance from the call team. Furthermore, it is anathema to comment that things seem relatively calm as evening approaches for fear of unlatching the gates of ER hell.

> One of our attending physicians refuses to touch his stringed instruments (guitar, mandolin) on call, believing that were he to start to play, he would be immediately summoned. Another won't go out to dinner. Another experiences palpitations in the shower because she swears she cannot set foot into one without the phone going off. Another always parked her car in the same spot on call days because it seemed to soothe the "call gods."

The phone sits on your belt or nightstand radiating malignant waves. Oddly, if it does not go off frequently enough, you will awaken with a myoclonic jerk, fumble for it, and test it to make sure it is fully functional. You may even call the hospital and ask if anyone has tried to call recently.

When the phone sounds, your physiology leaps into a "fight or flight" sympathetic overdrive. You bolt out of bed, chest tight, breathing labored, and heart pounding. You try to make sense of the conversation despite having gone from deep sleep to wakefulness in a millisecond. If you discern that you are not immediately needed, you collapse back into the bed, wide-eyed and unable to sleep for the next hour, as the cell phone continues to radiate pure evil.

Above all else, call is invasive. If you are like most physicians, you compartmentalize your life. You pour yourself into the workday but escape for a few hours at night and on weekends to a softer, gentler (and better smelling) world not so full of urgency, crisis, death, and tragedy. Call will have none of this. It inserts itself into every aspect of your life away from work and medicine. Meals, activities, time with friends, family gatherings, exercise, intimacy—nothing is sacred or is spared from invasion and interruption.

Here's what's interesting about the call psychology: Most physicians report that they don't mind the interruptions and invasions of call *if they are summoned for problems that truly require their services and expertise.* It is when they are called for trivial matters that they start to burn.

It is the rare individual who can deal with all the components of call without some degree of anger and, at times, unbridled rage. For example, when a physician facing a morning docket of 30 clinic patients is called at 3:00 a.m. about an inpatient who is having trouble sleeping civility becomes a true challenge. I (G. Simonds) can remember so many nights seething with rage about being called in to the emergency room for "trivial problems" or to soothe a doc's litigation paranoia ("patient cleared by neurosurgery").

Anger on call becomes reflexive. Many requests for assistance are bona fide and necessary, but many more tend to be trivial. Few physicians maintain utter civility over the years, after thousands of "nonsense" calls. They come to assume that all incoming calls will be nonsense and approach the call-back with thinly veiled hostility and righteous indignation. Any push-back on the other end of the phone may result in "melt-downs" and "blow-ups." Compounding matters, the angry physician has even more difficulty returning to sleep.

The psychology of call affects everyone who comes in contact with the physician.

> *Even my (G. Simonds) dog is affected! He senses when I am on call, and skulks around the house looking for places to hide when the phone inevitably goes off. When my children were young, they, too, sensed the malevolent air and steered clear. My whole family adopted the mindset that too much of a good thing would precipitate calls. Family activities thus became sedate, quiet, and passive. I always felt a bit of a leper—as the wife, children, and dog tip-toed silently about the house keeping distance between themselves and me.*

Remember also the chronicity of call. The typical physician may be on call every two to five nights for months, then years, then decades. For some, every night on call is sleepless. For those who sleep, their sleep cycles are likely ruined due to repeated interruptions or anticipated inter-ruptions—they sleep in effect with "one eye open." It is no wonder that many physicians devolve away from the pursuit of happiness in any form on call, only to settle into a state of suspended animation.

> *An endovascular specialist reported that she was on "stroke call" every other night. She had to rush to the hospital for a "stroke busting" procedure ap-proximately only four times a month. Nonetheless she absolutely could not fall asleep on stroke call nights. This began to significantly affect her physi-cal and mental health.*

Another seldom acknowledged phenomenon of the on-call experience is loneliness. The physi-cian on call faces the world alone. They head into the hospital along dark, barren roads, traipse down dimly lit, empty hospital corridors, and pass uninhabited nurses stations. Hospitals past 9:00 p.m. often resemble ghost towns, particularly on weekends. It is a lonely experience, and most physicians who take a lot of call relate feelings of profound isolation along with the other range of associated on-call emotions.

Residents and Call

For those of you who are still residents, your call is generally frequent and exceptionally busy. Yes, you get to go home by noon the next day, and this is a huge step in instilling some humanity into your training. But it still isn't easy. Systems with resident call coverage significantly lower their thresholds for summoning physicians. Thus, they will call you for any matter you could ever imagine, from the most dire to the supremely trivial.

> *A resident we know was summoned at three in the morning to the vascular floor because a patient complained of tongue pain. The resident racked her brain for a vascular-related differential diagnosis of tongue pain. When she went to see the patient, the nurse told her that the patient had been complaining about the tongue pain for a week but "none of the 'day doctors' had paid any attention," so she called the "night doctor."*
>
> *Another resident was called to renew a two-week standing order for patient restraints—at three in the morning.*
>
> *Another was called at 3:30 a.m. for a sleeping pill for a patient who was sound asleep but had complained the night before about a history of insomnia.*
>
> *Another resident was recently paged at 2:00 a.m. and asked whether he was the appropriate physician to call for problems in a post-operative patient. The resident answered in the affirmative and queried what was wrong with the patient. The nurse replied that nothing was wrong, and the patient was sleeping comfortably, but she wanted to know who to call if a problem were to develop.*
>
> *Another was called at 3:00 in the morning because a patient complained of foot itching. The resident prescribed an anti-fungal. Half an hour later he was called again and asked: "Remember the patient I called about with the itching? Well, it turns out he was not on your service—can you cancel the order please?"*

You can't make this stuff up!!

Combine sleep deprivation, a sense of being misused/abused, and the relentlessness of it all, and it is understandable that many of your colleagues feel victimized. Rather than leading to enhanced esteem and efficacy, call more typically leads to learned helplessness and loss of motivation.

Furthermore, even if you go home at noon the next day, a mere nap will not mend your sleep deficit. Sleep cycles don't work that way; you simply cannot catch up for a lost night's sleep by catching a few Zs the next afternoon. In fact, if you sleep too much in the afternoon, you won't be able to sleep that night.

Here are a few questions for you to contemplate and discuss with your peers, friends, families, mentors, or perhaps a therapist. Please see www.studergroup.com/thriving-physician for more questions.

Consider and Discuss

- What is your personal mental state on the day preceding a night of call? How about the day after?

- Are there any aspects of being on call that you enjoy? Sort of? Why?

- What is the perspective of the person calling you in the middle of the night? Are they trying to annoy you? What are they really looking for?

- How does call affect your family? Your friends? Your dog?

- What do you achieve by being righteously indignant when dealing with those who call you?

- If call is such an evil, how would *you* change medicine to obviate it?

Building Resilience

Call is a necessary burden in medicine, and this is unlikely to change drastically for the foreseeable future. Accepting this and accepting that it will be somewhat painful are steps in the right direction. Resistance only ratchets up your negative feelings. Instead, seeking solace from the fact that you are indeed serving a critically important purpose may help. Disease and trauma do not stop at sundown. People are in need, and you are there to help. It is a laudable calling.

- Try not to get wound up in the circumstances behind a belated consultation while on call. Yes, you may have been pulled into the care of a patient late at night after a Rube Goldberg string of mistakes and miscues, when ideally you would have been summoned during daylight hours, but fuming won't change the circumstances. Forget them and focus on the needs of the patient.

- No matter how trivial the issue, seek to bring comfort and reassurance to the patient.
- Try keeping a log of how many times you actually have helped someone when you were on call.
- Remind yourself that the trivial problems aren't so trivial to the patients. Nor, frankly, are they so trivial to the healthcare workers who are requesting your assistance.
- Challenge the confirmation bias. Is it really true that *every* time you seek some pleasure whilst on call you are called into the hospital? Keep track. If it is true, you probably have a legitimate argument for greater resources and more people taking call—or more time off at least.
- Try not to treat a call into the hospital as a tragedy for you and your loved ones. Allow everyone to recognize that you are helping people in distress when you have to break off a game of Monopoly, or a game of catch, with your kids. Sharing the sense of honorable duty and dedication dampens the disappointment and disseminates pride amongst your family members.
- Enlist your loved ones in your "mission." This lessens their distress about call and soothes their concern for you. Share with them stories of good things that resulted from your being on call—a diagnosis made, a family comforted, a life saved.
- Make a game of the call experience with your children. Hold lotteries on how many calls you receive, how many times you have to go in, how many patients you see, how much sleep you get.
- Greet everyone you encounter on call with politeness. Start with the original phone call. Force a smile and maintain a pleasant demeanor. Thank the caller for their concerns and ask if there is anything else you can do: "How else can I help you and our patient?" This will feel forced at first but will become easier over time. You will be pleasantly surprised at the results. People will get to know you as the sweet, helpful doctor and will actually seek to protect you. Let someone else be the angry, unhelpful, unpleasant one.

CHAPTER FIVE

Stop for a Moment!!!

Tell the truth: Have you spent any time reading and contemplating the questions in the "Consider and Discuss" section of each chapter and on www.studergroup.com/thriving-physician web page? If you haven't, you really should.

These questions get to the heart of your experiences, and the heart of your responses to them. We do not claim to hold all or any of "the answers" to how you can not only survive but *flourish* during your arduous, soul-sapping, mile-a-minute, insanely demanding medical day. But we can help you explore the challenges and find your own answers.

So, when you get to the questions, take a cleansing breath, read them, and *think*! A malady of a medical career is the "hurry sickness" that compels you to speed thoughtlessly through life. You buckle into that rocket sled on the first day of medical school, and next thing you know, you're at your retirement party! Our questions are designed to help you slow down and give voice to the thoughts and feelings bouncing around your cerebrum.

Medicine demands constant reflexive action on your part. Taken to the extreme, you can lose yourself in it all. We want you to periodically refocus on yourself. Re-identify your values, your person, your joys, your fears, your goals and aspirations. We hope that the questions and the process of considering them will blaze a trail back to you. The better you know you, the more likely you will be able to withstand the challenges of this crazy experience.

This takes both intention and courage. Some of what we discover when we stop and introspect is unpleasant or even a bit scary. Some is renewing, even exhilarating. Some questions may just help you find your best path or help someone else with theirs.

So please, read the questions, think, contemplate, and meditate. And think of your own questions; notice your own insights. Write them down, along with your thoughts, responses, and observations. Share your observations with us, with your comrades, or with friends and family.

CHAPTER SIX

ZZZZZ

Sleep Deprivation and Sleep Deficit

"The woods are lovely, dark and deep. But I have promises to keep and miles to go before I sleep."

—Robert Frost

"…Sleep deprivation is an illegal torture method outlawed by the Geneva Convention and international courts, but most of us do it to ourselves."

—Ryan Hurd

As a resident or practicing physician, long hours, call, home study, hyper-caffeination, and catching up on activities of daily living will deprive you of your much-needed sleep. This sleep deficit will be both acute and chronic in nature. Two-thirds of American medical residents reported sleeping fewer than six hours, even on nights when they are not on call, with one in five sleeping fewer than five hours.[1]

Sleep deprivation has emerged as a major risk factor for a number of chronic diseases and has repeatedly been correlated with decreased cognitive performance, increased likelihood of medical error, and higher instances of self-injury such as needle sticks.[2]

Being sleepy is one of the surest ways to underperform at work. A recent study of young physicians found that following one night of disturbed sleep there was a 25 percent drop in cognitive performance. Two nights of sub-par sleep resulted in an amazing 40 percent dip in cognitive performance.[3]

Our own research with residents found that self-reported sleep deprivation correlated with burnout, career dissatisfaction, and marital dissatisfaction.[4] And, with practicing physicians, whether we study work stress, maladaptive behavior, burnout, career dissatisfaction, psychiatric symptoms, or a physician mate's dissatisfaction with their marriage, physicians' reported levels of sleep loss and fatigue appear to both correlate with, and directly cause, these unwanted consequences.[5]

The perils to work performance that come with physician sleep deprivation are well-documented:

- Cognitive performance after 24 hours without sleep dips to the equivalent of performing with a blood alcohol level of .10.[6]
- In laparoscopic simulator performance studies, sleepy surgeons commit 20 percent more errors and take 14 percent longer to successfully complete tasks than their rested colleagues.[7]
- Compared to other times of day, fatigued physicians make medication errors 2.5 times more frequently between the hours of 4:00-8:00 a.m.[8]
- Medical interns who have gone 24 hours without sleep were demonstrated to sustain a 61 percent increased incidence of self-inflicted needle sticks, a 168 percent increase in motor vehicle accidents, and a 460 percent increase in motor vehicular near-misses.[9,10]
- Chronically sleep deprived individuals have four times the chance of catching a cold and 15% greater risk of experiencing and/or dying from a stroke.[11,12]

Sleep deprivation erodes your health and well-being. Chronic sleep deprivation leads to many potential somatic, functional, and emotional problems: overeating and weight gain, irritability and quick temper, loss of focus and concentration, diminished fine motor skills and exercise tolerance, loss of critical-thinking and decision-making ability, increased reaction times and decreased coordination, lack of motivation and depressed mood, blunted immune response, decreased visual acuity, poor memory registration and long-term memory recall, diminished executive functions and judgment, emotional lability or blunting, and more. It can even diminish your physical attractiveness through dehydration, pallor, dark circles, wrinkling, blotchiness, and, probably most importantly, loss of a smile.

The fact that patients require 24-hour-a-day care means sleep loss is inevitable for most physicians. Night-time coverage responsibility is generally shared between groups of specialists. Some specialties, like emergency medicine, break up the workweek into shifts that can lessen the impact of sleep loss. But no matter how shifts are arranged, a portion of the team will necessarily work through the night. And, just as circadian rhythm adjusts to a rotation of night call, moving back to day shifts begets yet another sleep adjustment. Some specialties try to mitigate the effects of sleep loss with work-free days following a night of call. But an afternoon nap will never make up for a lost night of sleep.

Many specialties still ascribe to an "old-school" approach to a lost night of sleep through call: a complete docket of work the following day. Night call can range from once a month for some physicians to every other night for others. Add to this stress cauldron the fact that trauma cases and so many other disease states seem to have a propensity to present at night.

> In studying our patient population at CC-VTC Neurosurgery, we found that 70 percent of our urgent and emergent consultations occurred between the hours of midnight and 6:00 a.m.

At many medical centers, night call can be very busy, even ferocious. Thus, in addition to robbing sleep, night call can cause profound physical, cognitive, and emotional fatigue.

Often, specialists in large tertiary care centers are bombarded with calls throughout a night to evaluate patients with problems that could easily be handled during daytime hours. In the modern medical center, however, the expectation is often for every patient to be evaluated immediately by the "appropriate" specialists. Patients may have been transported from long distances—sometimes for the most trivial of problems. EMTALA laws make it illegal to refuse transfer of patients from one center to another of higher level of care, no matter the reason. Frustration and resentment are thus heaped upon sleep loss and fatigue.

Making matters worse in hospitals with residents, there seems to be an inevitable night call "mission creep." That is, a "hair-trigger" develops for summoning resident assistance throughout the night. Residents are expected to expeditiously adjudicate even the most trivial of issues. When resident response is not immediate and definitive, they are routinely subjected to barrages of repetitive paging ("hammer pages"), berating, invective, and fights over patient admission. We experimented with this concept:

> *One of our attending neurosurgeons began taking primary neurosurgery call (with no resident buffer) once a week. We compared call experiences between the attending neurosurgeon and the residents. Phone call frequency was markedly less for the attending (an average 14 per night for the attending, 38 for the residents). Conflicts were limited, and the quality of phone consultations were distinctly better. Nurses were noted to hold many low-acuity calls to the morning. Some nurses and ER physicians actually stated: "I am so sorry; I would not have paged if I had known that it was an attending on call."*
>
> *We then "tricked" the system. We listed a resident on call and forwarded the resident's phone to the attending. The frequency of calls immediately increased, and quality of consultations plummeted.*

The sleep deprivation, and physical, cognitive, and emotional fatigue inflicted by nights on call require real restorative rest and repair. But for many physicians, any break or chance to rest waits until the following evening. Many physicians don't feel "normal" again until they have managed two nights of solid rest and sleep. This battery of sleep loss and whole-being exhaustion can be a routine part of your life for decades.

No matter how little sleep you think you need, you will routinely experience a full dose of sleep deficit. It is a rare individual who can regularly sustain fewer than seven hours of sleep a night without significant cognitive and emotional fall-out. Your body will scream for sleep. You will sleep at a moment's notice—during a lecture, working on a computer, sitting down at a meal, even standing and assisting in an operation.

> *One of our general surgery colleagues recounts an incident during his intern-ship where he fell so soundly asleep while standing and holding small retrac-tors in a parathyroid operation, he actually began dreaming. He then awoke with a myoclonic jerk. This made the operative field jump several inches. To his relief, the chief of surgery, a known "resident-slayer," took pity and turned to the circulating nurse, saying: "Nurse, go get Dr. Smith some NoDoz," and proceeded on with the surgery.*

Sleep will always win out. It is like a storm surge that runs up against a levy, finds a breach, and comes pouring through. Fighting it is futile and excruciating. You will ruin several evenings with your significant other collapsing into coma prior to a planned event. Or, you will go for a night out and try so hard to convey rapt attention to, and interest in, your date, only to find your eyelids getting heavier and your head nodding like a bobble-head doll. You will almost certainly fall asleep behind the wheel of your car at some point—hopefully for only a millisecond.

> *One of our physicians described his method of preventing falling asleep while driving home to D.C. after nights on call during a residency rotation at Maryland's Shock Trauma Center in Baltimore: "I would pack my mouth with as much gum as it could hold so that if I started to nod off—I would choke on the gum and awaken."*

Obviously, this is not our recommended solution! Parenthetically, be aware that many states now have laws that make you liable for accidents caused by your falling asleep at the wheel. So please don't even try to drive when you are carrying a significant sleep deficit.

A caveat: You may be able, to some degree, to counteract the detrimental effects on perfor-mance brought on by sleep deprivation through conditioning. In our lab, we ran a study of decrement in fine motor performance, cognitive function, and mood, in response to 24 hours of neurosurgery call. We found that subjects who were accustomed to sleep deprivation showed no decrement in any of these functions. "Unseasoned" subjects showed deterioration in all these functions. This in no way mitigates the solid cannon of evidence that chronic sleep deprivation is harmful on all fronts, but does suggest that we should be careful about shielding our trainees too much from the ravages of call and its inherent loss of sleep.

Here are a few questions for you to contemplate and discuss with your peers, friends, families, mentors, or perhaps a therapist. Please see www.studergroup.com/thriving-physician for more questions.

Consider and Discuss

- How do your friends, family, and significant others react when you fall asleep at inappropriate times and occasions? How does this make you feel?

- What are the circumstances that lead you to sleeping your best?

- How often do you compromise sleep to add more hours to the waking day? How many hours do you cut out?

- Do you awaken in the middle of the night and think about work? What do you think about? How does it affect returning to sleep? Do you ruminate? Can you stop the "thought train"?

- Is it wrong to sneak in a nap at work?

- Have you ever dozed off behind the wheel? On a date? During a patient interview? At an important meeting?

Building Resilience

- Consider making scheduling changes to facilitate better sleep habits. Researchers have suggested that physician sleep deprivation would be curbed by scheduling work patterns to allow every physician at least four hours of constant "anchor sleep" per night, a technique that has been shown to maintain a consistent 24-hour cycle of sleep and wakefulness and to reduce fatigue.[13,14]

- Take a midday nap of 10-30 minutes (longer is not beneficial). A short, midday nap was found to improve cognitive functioning and alertness among first-year internal medical residents.[15] Parenthetically, Winston Churchill swore by this technique in reducing his sleep needs to just a few hours a night throughout World War II.

- Avoid extended midday naps. They will disrupt sleep that night.

It is not uncommon for your sleep to become dysfunctional in a medical career even when you have ample time for it. This can compound your chronic deficit and can be insanely frustrating. If you find you are having difficulty with sleep despite being chronically tired, consider the following:

- If you feel yourself drifting off to sleep while relaxing in the evening well before bedtime, get up and move about to avoid disrupting your sleep cycle.
- Avoid using any chemicals to promote sleep (other than a warm glass of milk). All come with "baggage."
- Generally, a cool, darkened room is ideal for sleep. Consider soft music or soft ambient sound to buffer other noises in your environment.
- Avoid red wines, oak-aged alcohols, rich cheeses, spicy foods, and preserved foods in the evening.
- Keep a sleep diary. Compare foods, activities, conditions of nights of good sleep versus bad.
- Don't try to resolve the problems of the day lying in bed. Rather, if you are lying in bed awake, meditate, try breathing exercises, and/or focus on pleasant/serene thoughts and scenarios.
- Respect the basics of sleep hygiene recommended by the National Sleep Foundation:[16]
  - Avoid caffeine and alcohol close to bedtime.
  - Exercise can promote good sleep. Vigorous exercise should be avoided in the evening. Take it in the morning or afternoon.
  - Do something to relax (like yoga or meditation) before bedtime.
  - Avoid eating large meals close to bedtime.
  - When possible, get exposure to natural light during the day. Natural light exposure helps maintain a healthy sleep-wake cycle.
  - To the extent possible, establish a regular relaxing bedtime routine.
  - Avoid engaging in emotionally upsetting conversations and activities before trying to go to sleep.
  - Associate your bed with sleep. It's not a good idea to use your bed to watch TV, listen to the radio, or read.
- Assess your risk of sleep debt using the same test that most sleep clinics around the country use when evaluating new patients—The Epworth Sleepiness Scale:

The Epworth Sleepiness Scale is used to determine the level of daytime sleepiness. A score of 10 or more is considered sleepy. A score of 18 or more is very sleepy. If you score 10 or more in this test, you should consider whether you are obtaining adequate sleep, need to improve your sleep regimen, and/or see a sleep specialist:

The Epworth Sleepiness Scale[17]

Use the following scale to choose the most appropriate number for each situation:

0 = would *never* doze or sleep

1 = *slight* chance of dozing or sleeping

2 = *moderate* chance of dozing or sleeping

3 = *high* chance of dozing or sleeping

Situation	Chance of Dozing or Sleeping
Sitting and reading	
Watching TV	
Sitting inactive in a public place	
Being a passenger in a motor vehicle for an hour or more	
Lying down in the afternoon	
Sitting and talking to someone	
Sitting quietly after lunch (no alcohol)	
Stopped for a few minutes in traffic while driving	
Total score (add the scores up) (This is your Epworth score)	

The Epworth Sleepiness Scale Key

1 - 6   Congratulations, you are getting enough sleep!

7 - 8   Your score is average.

9 and up   Seek the advice of a sleep specialist without delay.

CHAPTER SEVEN

Risky Business

Conducting High-Risk Interventions

"The way to develop self-confidence is to do the thing you fear and get a record of successful experiences behind you. Destiny is not a matter of chance, it is a matter of choice; it is not a thing to be waited for, it is a thing to be achieved."
—*William Jennings Bryan*

"Opportunity dances only with those on the dance floor."
—*Anonymous*

Modern medicine is rife with interventions and procedures that risk horrific complications. Essentially every spinal surgery risks paralysis. Chemotherapies for cancer drive patients' systems to the brink of collapse in hopes of killing the cancer but not the host. Endoscopies can result in perforations with devastating consequences. You cannot watch a pharmaceutical commercial without being bombarded with an interminable list of potentially associated horrifying complications.

Many interventions and procedures walk a thin line between a good outcome and disaster. In resecting a malignant brain tumor, for example, the surgeon knows that the closer to a 99 percent tumor removal, the better the patient's long-term prognosis. Yet, the greater the volume of tumor resected, the greater the chance of significant neurological deficits. Anesthesiologists and emergency medicine physicians routinely push paralytic medications that halt spontaneous breathing in order to secure an airway or help failing ventilation—"securing" said airway is not always a "gimme," yet failure is a catastrophe for the patient.

Often, all the studying, testing, planning, and technological support in the world cannot anticipate or obviate catastrophic results. Equally often, on-the-spot decisions may save or lose a life. Exquisitely refined cognitive and technical skills and overall specialty-related acumen need to be developed over many years. And after long training periods, most physicians continue to hone and refine even the simplest of interventions throughout their careers.

When they begin to feel the strain of repeated high-risk care scenarios, physicians react in various ways. Some limit practice to less challenging "cases." Others sub-sub-specialize, to master a small subset of the cannon of their specialty, so as to avoid a broad array of pathologies. Some physicians bravely wade into the fray, fearlessly taking on the highest risk patients, only to be "rode out of town on a rail" because of high complication rates. On the other hand, some give up certain procedures after just one bad outcome.

Inevitably, and periodically, *you* must launch therapeutic interventions or perform procedures that test every ounce of your knowledge base, judgment, grit, adaptive intelligence, visual-spatial perception, and/or fine motor dexterity. Poor performance means devastation for the patient.

The preparation, execution, and follow-up for a single therapeutic intervention or procedure takes tremendous energy and focus. And this will be repeated several times a day, day after day.

> *One senior resident observed, "It would be nice if, every once in a while, after one of these super high-risk interventions or after a major unexpected complication, we could just sit down, think, discuss, rehash, review, dissect. But it seems that all we do is take a deep breath, gird our loins, and wade into an even bigger case. Shouldn't we savor the cases that go well and soothe ourselves after those that don't? But we never do…"*

Here are a few questions for you to contemplate and discuss with your peers, friends, families, mentors, or perhaps a therapist. Please see www.studergroup.com/thriving-physician for more questions.

Consider and Discuss

- What is the effect of multiple challenging patients or procedures in a row, or multiple complications in a row, on your psyche? What do you do to soothe the strain?

- Are there cases that strike fear in your heart? Which ones? Why? How could you change this? What are your physiological responses to such cases?

- How often do you over-test your patients despite your gut telling you that it is unnecessary? What drives this?

- What is worse—causing a bad outcome in a complex case or a simple case? Why?

- Does your system "get it" when you are caring for super high-risk patients? Are expectations changed? How do you change your expectations of yourself?

Building Resilience

When taking on high-risk interventions, it is best to be blatantly honest with yourself. Are you truly the right one for this job? Are there those who are far better suited for the intervention than you? If you can think of someone else who can take care of the situation substantially better than you, it is better to release the case than to face the psychological blitzkrieg of biting off more than you can chew.

On the other hand, remember that patients are depending on you to take some risk, and, at times, considerable risk. Taking no risk will often result in injury, progression of disease, or even a patient's demise. Without risk, no surgery would be possible; no medicine could be given. Sometimes you must power through your concerns about risk for your patients. There is strength in numbers, however. You don't always have to be a lone cowboy taking on the disease; enlist your colleagues when feasible.

At our program, we encourage faculty surgeons to operate together on high-risk procedures. That way, the most appropriate surgeon for the procedure can be involved in the case, and the acumen of the less-experienced surgeons can be enriched. The practice assures patients that they will have multiple opinions available during their surgeries and the skill of two full-fledged surgeons invested in their care. If a procedure starts to "wander off the tracks," there are two skilled surgeons working to get it positively redirected.

So much of medical intervention is thus a calculated risk. Are the benefits of this intervention better than the risks of leaving the disease process on its own recognizance? The answers are not always clear. The murkier it gets, the more risk you must be prepared to take. At times, you must take substantial risk for limited gain. It is even more gut-wrenching because you are taking the risk for someone else. But someone must take the risk and shoulder the burden of interventions that result in failure. Everyone cannot retreat into a shell of handling only simple cases and making only straight-forward decisions. High-risk patients need our help!

- If you routinely face high-morbidity/mortality situations, learn to "protect your professional flanks" (as well as your psyche). Document more extensively than normal the thought process behind your management, your counseling of the patient, your intervention, your follow-up. Make clear your understanding of the indications, risks, and benefits of your therapeutic intervention and the patient's comprehension of it. Importantly, document clearly the patient's co-morbidities and extenuating circumstances that ratchet up the risk of the intervention. The purpose here is to demonstrate your grasp of the gravity of your administrations, the profound acuity of the medial situation, and your thoughtfulness about it all. A high complication rate can be countered by solid data of increased patient acuity and demonstration of a well-reasoned and non-cavalier approach.

- No matter what, you must take good care of yourself. Relentless, unremitting exposure to high-risk scenarios wears on you, even if you are a bona fide adrenaline junkie. So establish breaks in the action. Take days off. Take lunch breaks. Escape from the pressure cooker now and then and distract yourself from ruminating over upcoming challenges.

- Be aware of your body's response to high-risk interventions, as there can be a very real element of physiological strain. This can have a bona fide detrimental effect on your physical health and should not be ignored. Watch for rapid heart rate, sweating, dry mouth, palpitations, tremor, etc. Work to relax and settle your overwrought physiology.

- Realize that when your physiology is on overdrive (sympathetic overload) it may be a warning that you are stretching. Reflect on the scenario and whether you are adequately skilled and prepared to face it. Perhaps the most effective way to overcome concern about risk is to develop *efficacy* for the task. Efficacy is task-specific self-confidence. Anything you can do to help you progress up the competency curve will help to quell your fear regarding that particular task.

- Get support along the journey. Engage trusted expert colleagues to help co-manage the sickest patients. Don't be afraid to go back to the books and dig into the knowledge base behind the situation you are facing. Knowledge here truly is power—power over related nervousness and anxiety. You will feel more competent and confident.

CHAPTER EIGHT

You Are What You Eat (and Drink)

Poor Nutrition and Hydration

"Life expectancy would grow by leaps and bounds if green vegetables smelled as good as bacon."

—*Doug Larson*

"If you don't take care of your body, where are you going to live?"

—*Unknown*

Physicians, and residents in particular, persistently demonstrate notoriously poor eating habits. This is a function of time and workload.

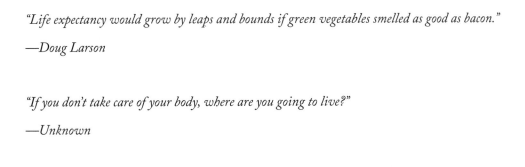

One of our medical colleagues reported eating, by necessity, the vast majority of his breakfasts, lunches, and dinners from vending machines—for the entirety of his SEVEN YEARS of training!

Modern hospitals have become somewhat better at making nutritious foods available, but these offerings take time to obtain and are generally more expensive than fast foods. Most require a trip to a busy cafeteria, which is anathema to the physician on the run.

As a physician, you are unequivocally prone to repeating vicious cycles that are right out of a nutritionist's nightmares. You choke down a sugar-infused breakfast (donut or muffin) as you head to "pre-rounds" with the ubiquitous coffee cup in hand. The diuretic effects hit as you head to the operating room or rounds, so you dash off to the bathroom. To prevent further bathroom breaks, you avoid liquids for many, many hours.

At some point, well past normal lunch time, you surface briefly from your work, parched and ravenous (thanks to a sugar- and caffeine-induced insulin release). You look at the clock and realize you have only minutes for sustenance. So you make a run for fast food, high in fats and carbohydrates. You guzzle down soda or fake fruit drinks—high in sugar content. Then, you are hit with the mid-afternoon doldrums. To fight off heavy fatigue, you ingest more coffee.

By evening, you are hypoglycemic and voracious again. You overindulge in hastily prepared dinners, often supplemented with alcohol as a sedative to counteract the recent caffeine. You then often turn to "comfort food" as an act of self-indulgence after a day of self-denial. Sitting on the couch downing high-sodium corn chips feels far more enticing than nibbling on celery between sets at the gym.

Poor nutrition and fluid intake carry a lot of baggage. Dehydration and serum glucose swings have both been tied to significant effects on mood, precipitation of depressed affect, agitation, anxiety, diminished concentration, and more. Dehydration in surgeons leads to a higher rate of kidney stones and DVTs. They are notorious for abstaining from any fluids after their first couple of cups of morning coffee to avoid needing breaks during their cases. Caffeine and alcohol disrupt already severely compromised sleep cycles. Eating too many high-calorie fast foods causes sluggishness, indigestion, and self-loathing. Dehydration and the ingestion of low-fiber foods lead to constipation and other G.I. ailments.

Further, you may be incredulous about the weight you are gaining (thus the self-loathing). Many of you will feel full, dyspeptic, and listless, which further discourages exercise. All of this becomes a self-perpetuating vicious cycle that can ultimately harm your body and spirit alike. To the outside world, it may seem ironic that we standard-bearers for the industry that has "health" right there in its name would be so *un*healthy. But anyone who works in the industry understands it perfectly.

Here are a few questions for you to contemplate and discuss with your peers, friends, families, mentors, or perhaps a therapist. Please see www.studergroup.com/thriving-physician for more questions.

Consider and Discuss

- How much time do you take for lunch and dinner on a typical day? Could you create more time?

- Do you feel compelled to diet? Why? How? How does a diet affect your mood and performance at work?

- What are several ways you can make it easier to maintain appropriate nutrition and hydration during a busy workday?

- What foods make you feel great? What foods make you feel bloated, sluggish, "fuzzy," anxious, or on edge?

Building Resilience

Like most of the resilience suggestions in this book, our suggestions here require *you* to put active thought and energy into your own well-being. Like an elite athlete, you push your body (and mind) to extremes at work. And like an athlete, you would benefit from a carefully selected diet. Take control of what you are putting into your body. A few pointers:

- Save the sodas and high-sugar drinks for a treat now and then. Drink water or diluted fruit juice and hydrate regularly. Keep a water bottle accessible through much of the day and take bathroom breaks when you need them.

- Seek balance in your food intake. Stay away from super-popular diets that have not been around for very long.

- Register how you feel after various foods and watch for overindulgence in unhealthy and unnatural substances.

- Enjoy a little of all food groups. It is okay to have a cupcake or some bacon now and then—but mix it in with lots of greens, vegetables, fruits, and nuts.

- Get into the habit of reading nutrition labels on all your foods. Pay particular attention to overall calories and sugar content.

- Make a concerted effort to reduce sugar intake. It is put into many foods without your realizing it.

- Limit dinners out and pre-prepared foods. These often have high sugar and fat contents.

- Stay away from white bread. Steer more to whole wheat breads and multi-grain breads.

- Grant yourself a few more minutes to eat the main meals of the day. Slower ingestion leads to smaller consumption. You deserve 30 minutes for lunch.

- Consider cutting your portion size by 1/4, 1/3, or even 1/2. You may combat some hunger for a while but soon you will adjust to the smaller allotments.

> *One of our colleagues told of how he looked in the mirror one day and was appalled at the bloated visage peering back at him. He stepped on the scale and had insidiously put on 30 pounds. For the next several weeks, he took any portion of food he had been served and cut it in half. He states: "At first, I was quite hungry on and off throughout the day. But then I started thinking, Unless you are truly starving, hunger is just a discomfort. And we physicians are used to discomfort on multiple levels—like loss of sleep, hours on our feet, etc. Why not treat hunger like any other discomfort?" He lost the 30 pounds in three months and stopped feeling the related hunger pangs within six weeks.*

- Rather than zone out in front of the TV with a bag of Fritos, take a walk around the neighborhood. This reduces your "snack-vulnerable" time. When you do settle down, purposefully set out something healthy: sliced apples, oranges, celery, nuts, etc.
- Discuss your diet with hospital nutritionists. (Even better, make it a sports nutritionist, if one is available.)
- Obtain a couple of up-to-date nutrition books. Look for athlete- or high performer-oriented books.
- Log an entire week of your own food intake, then review the nutritional value of your diet.
- Make a competition with your colleagues and coworkers to see who can eat the healthiest, most balanced diet over a week. (Everyone loves to compete!)
- Scout out the healthiest food services available in the hospital.
- Bring in healthy snacks to work. This will help you say no to the snack machine or the box of doughnuts a coworker brought in.
- Identify your ideal weight, then perform intermittent "weigh-ins." Reward yourself for making ground toward your ideal weight.
- Consider conducting cholesterol and blood sugar screenings.
- Attend healthy diet cooking classes.
- Reward yourself with desserts, chips, or candies *only* if you have logged in a set amount of exercise that day. And keep the quantity limited.

CHAPTER NINE

Your Worst Nightmare

The Torment of Bad Outcomes

"If you can meet with Triumph and Disaster
And treat those two impostors just the same...."

—*Rudyard Kipling*

"No matter what measures are taken, doctors will sometimes falter, and it isn't reasonable to ask that
we achieve perfection. What is reasonable is to ask that we never cease to aim for it."

—*Atul Gawande*

Physicians intervene medically because we believe that doing so will help patients, not harm them. But medicine is not a field of uniformly stellar outcomes. Due to the frailty of the organism, the aggressiveness of the disorders affecting it, and the nature of modern medical interventions themselves, patients frequently fare more poorly than we would wish. And this may occur far more frequently than we wish. For the physician at a busy tertiary center (or involved in one of many high-acuity specialty fields), bad outcomes may come "fast and furiously."

The fallout of bad patient outcomes needs to be anticipated and respected. To a degree, you can ascribe the majority to the nature of the presenting situation (e.g., it is hard to salvage a decent outcome in the case of a dominant hemisphere basal ganglia hemorrhage or a massive myocardial infarction). But each of us must also face the haunting question: *Have I contributed to the misery of my patient through my administrations or lack thereof?*

On occasion, our interventions leave patients hurt (new neurologic deficit, small M.I., painful joint, etc.), horrifically injured (renal failure, congestive heart failure, coma, hemiplegia, blind, etc.), or dead. This can even occur in a patient who undergoes a therapeutic intervention for a minimally symptomatic problem (atrial fibrillation ablation, anticoagulation for small stroke, brain tumor resection, abdominal aneurysm repair, etc.). In other words, a patient may walk into a hospital for an intervention and leave dead—or worse (yes, even worse than dead).

This is a burden few other people on earth face in their daily jobs. Your patient needs help and is trusting that you will bring him or her through his or her ordeal.

> *At the time of this writing, I (G. Simonds) had been made acutely aware of the miserable sting of a bad patient outcome. I removed an arteriovenous malformation that had bled from the cerebellum of an otherwise healthy elderly man. He awoke from surgery in good shape; however, an hour later, he rapidly deteriorated to coma. A CT scan demonstrated unexplained severe cerebellar swelling. We rushed him back to surgery and he survived, but unfortunately will likely not fully recover.*

Every bad outcome comes along with a dose of culpability for the managing physicians. Was the outcome due to "an act of God," the result of laziness (physical or intellectual), a minor error or a string of minor errors, a major mess-up, the end point of a combination of the natural course of the disease and a constellation of co-morbidities, medical ignorance or lack of skill, or bad luck? Was it an amalgam of all of these? In many ways, it doesn't matter; most physicians will feel some level of culpability for not doing better.

The National Academy of Medicine believes that thousands of patient deaths a year are the result of medical errors.[1] In response, massive patient safety and quality initiatives have been launched across the country. The resounding message is that many bad outcomes in patient care are indeed due to our mistakes. So, if we don't feel guilty enough for bad outcomes, we have the federal government joining the Greek chorus of woe.

Colleagues of ours note a shared response to a major complication in any of their patients (no matter the actual cause). They describe feeling as if everyone they encounter in the hospital hallways can clearly see a "Scarlet 'C'" (for COMPLICATION) tattooed upon their chests. They replay the related intervention in their heads nightly upon going to bed; they experience physiological responses (nausea, palpitations, sweats, stomach cramping) to any thought or reminder of the intervention. They state that they experience a form of survivor guilt, asking themselves, Why am I okay and the patient is devastated? *They ruminate on thoughts of inadequacy, ineptitude, and stupidity. They often don't begin to get over the effects of the complication until the patient leaves the hospital, or another major bad outcome occurs (thus sometimes swinging from one bad event to another).*

The emotional toll of bad outcomes can sideline a physician's career. Some physicians begin to contract, curtailing various services, withdrawing from high-level care, and sub-specializing to treating pathologies of less acuity.

If the onslaught is particularly vicious and repetitive, or if the physician does not have the psychological makeup to absorb the repetitive insults to the psyche, he or she may contemplate full retreat to retirement, change in career, or strict limitation of services to low-risk procedures and non-urgent conditions.

No one is immune to repetitive bad outcomes. Too much, and a sense of futility, nihilism, and learned helplessness will creep in. On the outpatient side, at least there are the uplifts of interacting with thankful patients who have come through severe illnesses and injuries. But on the inpatient side, you have the *Groundhog Day* phenomenon of experiencing wave after wave of hopelessly ill patients, and bad outcomes after bad outcomes, which will take its toll over time.

Here are a few questions for you to contemplate and discuss with your peers, friends, families, mentors, or perhaps a therapist. Please see www.studergroup.com/thriving-physician for more questions.

Consider and Discuss

- Must you always be perfect? What is your definition of a "good enough" performance today?

  Example: "I consider it a good enough day if _____."

- How do you handle making significant mistakes?

- Do you feel emotionally stronger or weaker now than you did at the start of your medical career? Why?

- How do you protect yourself from caring too much about the patients and their outcomes?

- Do you perceive every bad outcome as a personal failure? If so, how can you tone this down?

- Do you tend to blame bad outcomes on everyone other than yourself? Is this realistic?

Building Resilience

Remember, if you intervene on the behalf of sick patients, you will have bad outcomes. The sicker the patients, the more frequent the bad outcomes. Even the not-so-sick patients will, on occasion, experience bad outcomes.

- Accept that you will make mistakes that hurt people. This is the reality of medicine. Those who maintain that bad outcomes can be totally avoided are not really "playing the game." If you cannot somehow incorporate this philosophy into your care, you run the risk of tearing yourself apart, particularly if you are in a high-risk field. This does not mean that you should ascribe every bad outcome to the "will of God," or bad luck, or the mysteries of the human body. Rather, you need to maintain an intellectual curiosity and honesty about all outcomes positive and negative, and a desire to improve outcomes at all times.

- Keep in mind that improving outcomes does not mean zero complications. Perfectionism will kill you. Perfect outcomes are a rarity in medicine. But you can always strive for *excellence*. Excellent care still involves complications and bad outcomes.

- Use every case as a learning opportunity; note what went wrong and what worked well. Often a "near miss" with a great outcome holds more lessons than a case of one mistake after another. And just because a case goes terrifically, it does not mean that you did everything right. Analyze your successes as well as your failures.

- Seek a healthy balance. Forgive yourself for complications and bad outcomes (which are inevitable), but subject yourself to healthy skepticism when it seems as if you can do no wrong. There is an interesting psychology surrounding outcomes. We tend to beat ourselves to pieces over bad outcomes, and elevate ourselves unjustifiably after good outcomes.

> A colleague of ours maintains that, "I am at my most dangerous after a string of great patient results. I begin believing I can take care of anything. I begin to choose my interventions poorly. I become rather cavalier. And then, man oh man, do I pay for it!"
>
> Another colleague related this story: "For my first year out of training, everything I touched turned to gold. I was performing procedures far beyond my training and experience, and they were turning out wonderfully. I began believing that I was truly superior, that I could do no wrong. I took on anything and stopped asking for help or advice. Then all hell let loose. It started with a young man from whom I successfully removed a pineal tumor—a big operation. Two days after surgery, though, he hemorrhaged into the resection bed and died. Several more major complications followed. It nearly ended my career. I could not fathom that I was not what I thought I was. Now I questioned if I was competent at all—whether it was right for me to continue being a surgeon."

- Accept that your fellow physicians (and all healthcare professionals) can have bad outcomes without being incompetent. The more you see yourself as a member of a team and a community that has to deal with these crushing challenges, the less alone you will feel.
- Rather than condemn colleagues for bad outcomes and complications (overtly or silently), realize what they must be going through and offer solace.
- Think "team." Great care is the product of teamwork. On the other hand, bad outcomes affect the whole team. Accept that seeking and offering support in the wake of a bad outcome is a survival skill that will serve you well throughout your life in medicine.

- Some extra compassion is due to you out there who practice in small groups or solo. To whom do you turn for support and compassion when the heartache of an unwanted outcome haunts you?
- Debrief your responses to a bad outcome with trusted colleagues and friends. The gory details of the complication are important to a morbidity and mortality conversation but less so to a debriefing. Rather, focus on your response and how you may work through the experience in a constructive and healthy manner.
- Share with others the methods of weathering the storm and returning stronger than before.

CHAPTER TEN

Hey, Guys, Watch This!!

The Self-Denial/Overindulgence Cycle

"Earth provides enough to satisfy every man's needs, but not every man's greed."
—*Mahatma Gandhi*

"Virtue itself turns vice, being misapplied,
And vice sometime by action dignified."
—*William Shakespeare,* Romeo and Juliet

You work like a fiend for several weeks straight and finally get a break. You head straight for the mall and buy a very expensive pair of shoes that you might wear only twice. The price tag takes a toll on your bank account, but you feel validated by the fact that you are one of the hardest working people in your hospital.

You weather a week of stat pages, bad complications, and a handful of patient deaths. You get home Friday night, make a martini (or maybe several!), and spend the rest of the weekend binge watching your favorite shows on Hulu. You tell yourself: *I earned this one.*

You just finished up a high-stakes, ten-hour operation that soaked up every bit of your focus, concentration, and technical skill. A recovery room nurse interrupts your charting and asks you for the patient's diagnosis. You bark: "Did you not bother to read the chart? Your *job* is to familiarize yourself with the patient, not bother the surgeon with stupid questions."

One pitfall of the extensive self-denial and self-sacrifice existence that is a medical career is the tendency to swing wildly to overindulgence once you are finally released from the grip of responsibilities. Examples are pervasive and often involve truly self-destructive behaviors that are usually justified with a notion like: *I work so hard and sacrifice so much, I owe it to myself to splurge a bit.*

These splurges are frequently over-the-top, expensive, and potentially habit forming. Physicians may justify periods of heavy drinking this way, or infidelity, or substance abuse, or other high-risk behaviors. The sense of release after prolonged denial may be quite intense, thus rewarding the self-indulgent behavior and making it more difficult to curtail. This type of "recursive" coping cycle is maladaptive and can lead to destroyed careers, lost friendships, financial ruin, and broken marriages.

Self-denial is a critical skill that every physician must master. You must be able to tolerate extended periods of ignoring and/or suppressing your own comforts, drives, and desires, in order to accomplish the daily mountain of work before you. Falling into subsequent self-indulgence, however, is all too easy. You may even engage in "try to top this" competitions with colleagues.

A couple of methods of self-indulgence are a little less obvious. Many physicians become excessively dedicated to work—that is, overindulgent in self-denial. They proudly work harder than any other colleague. During this "zealot" stage, they take more call, sit at the patient's bedside all night (when not necessary), stay in the hospital for days at a time, and/or go without food or hygiene.

Such self-denial may become addictive, and it leads to irritability, withdrawal, and rumination. The physician may become detached and overly perfectionistic and insist that others behave professionally more like him/herself. Besides being insufferable, these physicians spiral downwards in this world of martyred self-denial, and their life outside the walls of the hospital withers. For many, this downward spiral settles into full-blown compassion fatigue, where, despite hanging around the hospital endlessly, the affected physician no longer is capable of feeling empathy or compassion for his/her patients and deteriorates in self-care.[1]

An even more common form of overindulgence is the violation of the "social contract" of civility and respect between coworkers. The physician feels entitled to lash out at subordinates for often arbitrary reasons. The physician justifies this as reasonable in that no one else has to work as hard, or bear the responsibilities, or make the tough calls, or take the risks, or make the decisions that he or she must. The history of medicine is littered with this behavior—even to the most outlandish of extremes (horrendous insulting and belittling, screaming tantrums, throwing equipment, even physical abuse).

It is surprisingly easy to drift into this type of behavior—even for nice physicians...even for you! You start merely by being distracted, in a hurry, non-communicative. Month by month you get a little more intolerant. You begin to normalize uncivil behaviors in yourself at work that you would never countenance in the outside world. You justify this because of the extremes you must suffer in the workplace. Next thing you know, you are cursing like a sailor and throwing things. Congratulations, your overindulgence has led you to become an insufferable jerk!

Here are a few questions for you to contemplate and discuss with your peers, friends, families, mentors, or perhaps a therapist. Please see www.studergroup.com/thriving-physician for more questions.

Consider and Discuss

- How do you feel in the aftermath of an unhealthy indulgence?
- What is your interpersonal reputation with your coworkers? Truly? Do coworkers "light up" when you walk onto the ward? *Do* you energize those around you?
- What activities of yours outside of the hospital are adaptive? That is, they bring you joy, health, happiness, fulfilment, energy, recharging?
- What activities of yours outside of the hospital are maladaptive? That is, they lead to potential problems for you?
- What are you owed for your intelligence, hard work, industry, bravery, years put-in, leadership, sacrifice, and delayed gratification?

Building Resilience

Remember, if you are going to sustain any real personal well-being, you must beware of and manage this cycle of self-indulgence. "I am owed this" is a magnificently dangerous sentiment and has led to disaster for literally thousands of physicians. It can be used to justify virtually any activity or behavior. We are not advocating for you to never indulge yourself. You are not a monk. Soothing your wounds, restoring your energy banks, and turning your mind to things other than medicine are all critical to your wellness.

- Be on the lookout for justifying potentially harmful indulgences with the notion that you owe yourself said activity.
- As for the "incivility" form of overindulgence, watch out! In regard to behavioral norms in hospitals, the tide is turning. Healthcare workers, particularly nurses, have had enough, and have established a whole new system of mores and expectations for *your* professional behavior. Unprofessional behavior is one overindulgence that simply will no longer be tolerated. If this is one of your overindulgences, you need to get it under control immediately.

> *We have seen more physicians lose their jobs over interpersonal professional behavior in the past five years than in the previous 30.*

- Scan the millions of positive indulgences that can lead to your own personal growth, health, and happiness—like those that connect you with others and those that bring you calm but also energize you.
- Try out many forms of healthy indulgence for size—always in moderation.
- Consider healthy indulgences such as learning to play an instrument, hiking, biking, learning a new language, reading, taking art classes, volunteer work, astronomy, gardening, recreational sports, etc. Try to cultivate a few so one activity doesn't become a fetish—one into which you sink all your energy, emotional resources, and money.
- When you are tempted to indulge in maladaptive behaviors, stop and ask yourself why you are doing this. What will you gain? What are the risks? Is it harmful to you or others? Are you proud of this activity? Is it some form of twisted competition with your colleagues? Is it illegal? Would your loved ones be hurt if they found out? Does it put your job at risk? Can any other activity provide the same positives with fewer negatives? If you proceed with the activity, ask yourself these same questions the next day.
- Write down all your current "extra-curricular" activities. Put those that are clearly positive and healthy on one side and those that risk being unhealthy for you on the other.

Consider each of the maladaptive activities. Can they be made more adaptive with modification or do they need to be thrown out?

- Do you have enough adaptive activities? If not, write down all the hobbies and activities in which you used to engage before you entered medicine. Are there any that are adaptive and would bring you pleasure now?
- Sample and list some of your friends' extra-curricular activities. Do any fit the bill?
- Imagine you are watching yourself in your day-to-day activities through a one-way mirror. Are you a pleasure to be around, or are you caustic, sarcastic, and/or abusive? Make an all-out effort to be the former. This way, even on a bad day you are less likely to stray into the worst behaviors (further to go), and more likely to be forgiven if you do.

CHAPTER ELEVEN

Families Are the Compass That Guides Us

The Stress That Accompanies Starting and/or Maintaining Family Relations

"The family is one of nature's masterpieces."

—*George Santayana*

Wife and child,
Those precious motives, those strong knots of love.

—*William Shakespeare,* Macbeth

Special thanks to Dr. Lola Chambless of Vanderbilt University Neurosurgery for providing much material and thoughtful analysis on the implications of pregnancy in medicine. Her lectures on the subject are eye-opening, informative, and riveting!

The decision to start a family is one that should not be taken lightly. Not only must you come to realize that you are ready to become a parent—which in and of itself is a massive life decision—but as a physician, you must prepare to add even more responsibility to an already full plate.

Balancing work and parenting is, of course, difficult for professionals in every industry. That's why so many highly educated men and women (singles *and* couples) are delaying parenthood or forgoing it all together. (Indeed, over the past few years, we've seen a spate of articles touting the benefits of the child-free lifestyle.) Yet for physicians, in particular, the brutal work hours, nights on call, and other effects of the avalanche of the unique stressors explored in this book can vastly complicate an already complicated life.

Don't get us wrong! The rewards of parenthood are profound and real, and we would never discourage anyone who wants children from having them. But being a parent *and* a full-time practicing physician is incredibly difficult, and it's not for everyone. And of course, on top of the work/life issues that plague prospective parents of both genders, women must also grapple with the issue of biology: It is the female resident or physician who must find the right time to procreate. Between her many years of medical training, which coincide with her prime childbearing years, choosing between competing priorities is difficult indeed.

According to a 2013 Gallup Poll of Americans aged 18-40, 74 percent had children and 19 percent wanted to have children.[1] The average American woman's first birth occurs at age 24. The average age of students entering medical school is now 24.5. The average American female surgeon's first birth is at age 34. Natural female fertility drops to 50 percent not long after the age of 35. Medical school is generally four years long, and residencies are trending to ever-longer durations, lasting anywhere from three to eight years. Do you see the potential challenge here?

The typical female medical student is firmly planted upon an educational conveyor belt for anywhere from seven to fourteen years. This, during the prime of her fertility. She will finish training at an age where fertility rates are dropping dramatically. If she is a neurosurgeon who goes on to a year of fellowship after training, for example, she won't begin her bona fide career until she is 36 to 38 years of age.

So, when's the best time for women in medicine to have their children? Should they give birth before the start of medical school? Should they face the disdain, guilt, discomfort, jealousies, snarky comments, risk, and super-fatigue of having children during their residencies? Or, do they hold off, risk the high infertility rates, and start their families during a period in their career where work and call demands may actually eclipse those of residency and while they are trying to build a practice, garner referral patterns, and establish networks?

The fall-out of this dilemma is tangible. The rate of pregnancy complications amongst female surgeons has been documented at 32 percent, compared to 15 percent for average U.S. women.[2] This is presumably because pregnant surgeons continue their harrowing work schedules up to the very last minute. Probably, many work even harder and longer hours, continuing to take on the significant physical and mental demands, in order to make up for anticipated lost contribution to the overall effort during their perinatal time away.

And what if all does not go perfectly? Consider the effects of a high-risk pregnancy where a mother may be instructed to "take it very easy" or to take to bed for months at a time. For many physicians, no extra support nor moderating of their work schedules is offered or even considered. In fact, any hint of such may engender deep resentment and denigration amongst their colleagues.

This dilemma is a tremendous unspoken stressor amongst a sizable portion of this generation of physicians. Keep in mind that 50 percent of medical school students are now women.[3] There is no perfect nor even optimal timing for pregnancy or maternity leave in a medical career. Most medical organizations are simply not built to easily absorb extended physician absences, whether for pregnancy, maternity leave, vacation, illness, injury, or any other reason. Anyone's extended absence requires others to add considerable work to their already heaping plates.

This is particularly pointed with respect to call coverage. A team that has been relatively comfortable with a one-in-five call night schedule can become heavily strained if the call drops to one-in-four and can implode if it drops to one-in-three. Thus, there is the potential for profound resentment and even overt hostility when a physician's prolonged absence from the work roster is perceived to be totally voluntary (i.e., as in a pregnancy or maternity leave).

Female physician acquaintances who became pregnant during residency and/or whilst in a group practice recount examples of boorish, outlandish, and shaming comments directed at them by supervisors, seniors, and colleagues (and/or by their colleagues' life mates!). Several recalled colleagues giving them the "cold shoulder" for months and even years after returning from maternity leave. Many reported crushing guilt while away, to the extent that they began taking call during leave and/or cut their leaves short. Many women we know returned to full-time work within TWO WEEKS after giving birth.

Men are beginning to feel the strain as well. They don't want to continue the legacy of absent physician parents. They too want to be part of the pregnancy and infancy experiences. Yet, if they dare take extended paternity leave, or alter their full-time work schedules, they, too, are met with subtle or blatant questioning of their commitment to the profession.

And, of course, the pull to home and hearth does not end on the last day of maternity/paternity leave. In fact, it intensifies logarithmically as the baby grows and develops, and as each new addition to the family arrives…including grandchildren! The feelings of longing and guilt on the part of the hard-working physician parent can be substantial if not overwhelming.

> *I (W. Sotile) have personally counseled thousands of male physicians who stated that leaving home before their young children awakened, and returning home after their bedtimes, was one of the toughest parts of their career.*
>
> *One of our colleagues recounted how his solution, much to his wife's chagrin, was to wake his young children up each night around 10:00, as he got home from the long work days of his residency.*

The simple truth is that a career in medicine is not conducive to participating in family life. The hours away are inordinately long. The days are physically and emotionally draining. The invasion of call is omnipresent. The work does not stop at the home's front stoop.

Challenges to the family structure compound throughout a medical career. Medical training takes the majority of physicians far from their "hometowns." Then, few find ideal practice opportunities in their chosen specialties that are situated near their extended families. Thus, generational lines and interactions are disrupted more in medicine than in most other professions.

Clinical medicine has been described as a "jealous mistress"—it certainly offers periods of significant pleasure and fulfilment, but it is always exacting and is relentlessly demanding. Try as you might to routinely walk away from it, it will quickly seize you back or preoccupy you.

All of our faculty are quite superstitious about taking real time off from work and fully engaging in family life. They recount examples of vacations disrupted by last-minute clinical disasters that required a few more days of work or hanging around in town. Many a vacation must be conducted under the pall of sadness, guilt, and ruminations about a bad patient outcome or a horrible complication.

For those in academic medicine and/or involved in political activity within their specialties, the work/family dynamic can be even more strained. The demands for writing, engaging in research, and frequent cross-country trips to various meetings, courses, and programs do not follow family-friendly schedules.

If you are like many physicians, you may long for a life where you don't have to feel ashamed for being pregnant or for making time to spend with your loved ones. Your longing to be with your family may strain your tolerance for what happens at work. Is your anger at a patient who arrives late for the last appointment of the day truly related to his being late, or is it related to your distress about missing your child's recital? Could your chaffing at an operating room's protracted "turnover time" actually be related to your sadness about missing your child's last high school soccer game? Could your frustration with your work schedule be related to deep unrest, as you witness all the "normal" families carrying on "normal" family activities?

Regardless of how you define "family," physician resilience requires that you deal head-on with a constant "double-bind": Should you be at home with your family or at work with your patients? There is no such thing as a balanced life. The balance will tip one way or the other, and for most physicians, generally in the direction of the work. If not managed mindfully, regret, guilt, and longing about missed family experiences will fill your psyche.

> *One of our faculty members was a multi-sport athlete throughout his early life. Despite the hundreds of games and meets in which he participated, it was not until his junior year in college that his father, a busy general practitioner, actually made it to one. This left an indelible impression. In response, our faculty member obsessively pushed and struggled to make as many of his own children's games, meets, and events as possible. This stress of getting there often dampened the potential enjoyment of the activity.*

Here are a few questions for you to contemplate and discuss with your peers, friends, families, mentors, or perhaps a therapist. Please see www.studergroup.com/thriving-physician for more questions.

Consider and Discuss

- How often do you spend substantial time with your parents, siblings, and extended family? How does it feel when you leave them?

- When is the right time to start a family in a medical career? What is needed from a parent for the ideal upbringing of children?

- How should maternity/paternity leave be handled in a medical practice? How should it affect physician reimbursement and promotion?

- What would be the absolute ideal work hours to promote a sensational career *and* family life?

- Should there be more physicians in your specialty to help "spread the load," such that you all have more time for your families and outside interests? What sort of salary reduction would be acceptable to afford you substantially more time at home?

- What do you owe your colleagues for missing months of work?

Building Resilience

Here we're going to discuss building resilience in two separate but related areas: pregnancy timing and work/family dynamics.

The Pregnancy Conundrum

Biologically speaking, there *is* an ideal time for pregnancy. That is when it is most healthy for the mother, the child, and the entire family. This can put it right in the middle of medical school, residency, and/or an early career, but so be it.

We have for so long skewed the perspective on this issue dramatically away from the rational and sensible (and not without a good dose of misogyny), that we have difficulty accepting a different approach.

- Recognize that for many people the drive to have children, and the fulfilment derived from doing so, is fundamental to the human experience. As a society, shouldn't we celebrate and support responsible parenthood, rather than throw every obstacle we can in the way?
- Know your organization's guidelines for maternal and paternal leave. Amazingly, until recently, our national accrediting bodies for medical schools and residency training programs had made no real provisions for pregnancy during the training years. This is likely because in previous generations the pregnant medical student, resident, or fellow virtually did not exist. Nearly all the trainees were male. And, of course, historically, little thought was ever given to any man's desire to help raise his children. Our accrediting and advisory bodies continue to be way behind on this. There is no built-in flexibility for extended absence, particularly in the residency world. In fact, this is true with respect for protracted absences of any kind (illness, family crisis, etc.).

The law has taken one step in the right direction. Maternity leave in any work setting is supported for up to 12 weeks through the Family and Medical Leave Act (for women *and* men). It is illegal for residents to be tasked with making up or "front-loading" lost work or call nights. Penalties for infraction, or for any sense of related prejudice, can be steep, and civil awards have been astronomical. In other words, residency programs, practices, and systems better get it: You are entitled to maternity leave without penalty or prejudice. Period.

> *National medical specialty bodies are getting it, too. Here is the 2016 state-ment from the American College of Surgeons: "The College recognizes that a successful surgical career should not preclude a surgeon's choice to be a parent…choosing to become a parent does not detract from one's full pro-fessional commitment as a surgeon."*

The environment is not perfect, but it is improving. We maintain that it is absolutely reasonable and healthy to plan pregnancies as they are desired and can be supported. In other words, **when you are ready**.

Ideally, your work/training system will be prepared to absorb your absence and will support your mental and physical health throughout the experience (and beyond). If in any way, prejudice is shown against you, know your rights and defend them.

- Discuss the possibility of pregnancy and subsequent maternity leave with your super-visors and employers well in advance. This would allow them to arrange coverage and support for you, and hopefully celebrate the process with you. This would also help you and your system "normalize" the concept that pregnancy and related absences are and will be part of the culture going forward—and that this is a good thing. If you are a family-devoted man, the same is true for you. You will have some cultural hurdles but recognize the intensely important role of support for your child's mother and your own interaction with your child.

The Work/Family Tightrope

Stress about juggling work and family is something that everyone in medicine shares. It is time for us to "normalize" a new culture with respect to time away from work.

- Start by normalizing for yourself the idea of routinely taking time to be with your family, to spend certain meals with them, to take periodic long weekends with them, to occa-sionally go on an extended vacation with them.
- Accept that work/life "balance" is a fallacy. Our multiple life roles leave us perpetu-ally "imbalanced." If we are prudent, we will learn to regularly bolster some life arena (family, work, self, primary relationship) that has atrophied a bit from inattention.

Accept, though, that there will always be an imbalance, often leaning in the direction of work.

- Remember that medicine needs your commitment and dedication. It does not need you as a burned-out remnant of what you once were. A key to your mental health is sustaining positive personal relationships. You need time and real interaction with your family to keep doing the amazing work you do. Both your home and work lives need to be in harmony, but either can bring the other down.

- Develop rituals that your whole family enjoys and set them in stone—be it nightly meals, Friday night board games, Saturday trips to the park, or Sunday hikes in the mountains.

- Now that medicine is generally practiced in teams, depend on your team to break free of work demands regularly. The better your team, the more you can depend on each other to cover one another. Remember, the more collaborative and collegial *you* are, the better your group will function as a team.

- Recognize that you will "short" your loved ones on many normal family activities. Be sure to make some recitals and sporting events, but don't try to over-correct and make them all (this is unrealistic). Let your children know you so greatly enjoyed watching them and that you were proud of their efforts!

- When you cannot make an event, have your child relive it with you when you return home. Demonstrate your keen interest and pride despite your absence. Fuel his or her interests with your interest. Be liberal with your pride in him or her.

- Counter the distress of what you miss by being mindfully present when you are with your loved ones. Be creative: Even the most mundane of activities can be elevated to the status of "quality family time."

> *A physician we know routinely says to each of his three children, "Spending this time with you will be (or has been) the best part of my day." He says this if he's carpooling them, putting them to bed, or simply eating their latest version of take-out dinner. Any activity will do! The message he is giving to his family is that, for him, being with them is an utter joy.*

- Never put forth that your career or even your patients are more important to you than your family, but do remind them that you have a duty to honor your job and your patients.

- Make your family a "medical family." Let them know that because they were so gracious in excusing you from a family activity, someone in distress was helped. Bring them to work on occasion and let them experience some of your world so it is all very real to them. This will help them understand and make peace with why you must periodically disappear.

- Help your life partner with the mundane chores of family life. A little can go a very long way. Enlist the children.

- It sounds so cliché but replace quantity with quality. Resist the temptation to collapse in front of the TV when you get home. Get creative with the limited time you have together. Capture the golden moments with your family. Keep a journal. Take lots of pictures. Then, on hard, lonely days at work, savor the images. They will be islands of peace, warmth, and sanity in your crazy, hectic world.

CHAPTER TWELVE

50.7 Percent: Women in Medicine

"Stop telling girls they can be anything they want when they grow up. It's a mistake. Not because they can't, but because it would have never occurred to them they couldn't."

—*Sarah Silverman*

Special thanks to CC-VTC Neurosurgeon Dr. Cara Rogers for greatly assisting us with this chapter.

We fully acknowledge that there is something ironic about two old men opining on the experiences and travails of women who have entered the field of medicine. That is why we made sure to seek help with this one from someone who "gets" these issues firsthand (see above)! We also acknowledge that people of *all* biological, cultural, and racial backgrounds have for far too long been subjected to mistreatment, bigotry, prejudice, injustice, harassment, and outright abuse at the hands of those of privilege and power within the field of medicine.

However, we have repeatedly been asked by our audiences to specifically address the plight of those who will soon make up over 50 percent of the physician workforce—women. And so, here we are. We suspect that, sadly, many of our female colleagues have already experienced many of the "stressors" we will discuss in this chapter. By bringing these uncomfortable dynamics and out-and-out bad behaviors into the light, we hope to play a small role in helping to accelerate the much-needed change that's already starting to take place.

Until very recently, medicine was a bastion of male egos, male dominance, and professional machismo. The entire language of medical exchange was peppered with fraternal references, sports analogies, misogyny, and not a little dosing of sexual innuendo. In these days of yore, yearly female entrance into any medical discipline could be measured in the single digits by percentage. Well, times have certainly changed. In 2017, for the first time, women outnumbered men in medical school, representing 50.7 percent of matriculants.[1]

So yes, the landscape of medicine is evolving (we would say belatedly, and for the better). This does not mean, however, that unique stressors do not persist for women in the field. In fact, women face significantly higher rates of depression and higher rates of attrition than do their male counterparts as residents and as practicing physicians. Work/life balance challenges are purported to be at the center of this disparity, but there is much more to it.

Certainly, the echoes of the male-dominated past still ring throughout the hallways of modern medical practice, particularly in certain subspecialties. Sadly, misogyny, subtle innuendo, unwanted advances, and overt sexual harassment have been part of the medical landscape for too long.[2]

Medicine creates a "perfect storm" for such behavior with its inherent hierarchies and readily demonstrable power differentials amongst the medical ranks. Men still often hold the most elevated positions in many a department, and they come into contact with wave after wave of young women trainees and colleagues whose career advancement depend on their support and cooperation. Although improving, the culture of many medical settings has yet to completely clear the vestiges of the *Mad Men* era of the discipline. In some arenas, female professionals are still subjected to inappropriate communications and behaviors. And harassment need not be overt to be corrosive. Subtle streams of inappropriate interaction are often tolerated for months or years, and the effects can be withering.

> *Personal interviews reveal that some female physicians are routinely exposed to a startling array of lecherous and misogynist behaviors. Some report feeling unsafe in certain corners of the hospital, particularly when on call at night. Sexualized and misogynist behaviors can be so common that some women physicians report becoming desensitized to it. Others report that it casts a pall on all male-female workplace interactions. Even "innocent" romantic advances can become grating and anxiety-provoking in such environments.*

What's more, unwanted courting behavior, misogyny, and over-sexualized interactions are not the sole purview of the medically powerful.

> *Some female physicians that we have interviewed report being subjected to sexualized comments, come-ons, and even fondling by janitors, food service personnel, aides, repairmen, security personnel, and even patients.*

Being subjected to repeated misogyny, innuendo, or sexual advances can be very damaging to your resilience. A sense of loss of control and powerlessness may become pervasive. You begin to feel isolated and victimized. A sense of profound loneliness may follow. Such an atmosphere may suck the joy right out of work for you and spill out into your home life.

> *Happily, many of the women physicians we have interviewed report a changing tableau in medicine. Many speak of a much less sexually charged and hostile atmosphere, and a greater willingness of colleagues to come forward and confront inappropriate behaviors, and to support one another.*

Even without the specter of harassment and misogyny, the dynamic between the sexes can be challenging in the heavily hierarchical medical workplace. Appropriate "courting" behavior in a professional setting may be difficult to define and codify. Most institutions have few, if any, guidelines on appropriate romantic/sexual behavior between employees. Some have zero-tolerance fraternization policies, even between colleagues of equal "rank."

The dynamic may be confusing for all and may potentially create an uncomfortable and/or threatening environment for many. When, for example, is it appropriate for coworkers to share a lunch or a drink out at a local restaurant? What if one party is a department chair and the other is a resident or a medical student? Is it acceptable to ask any coworker out on a date? When do repeated requests for a date become harassment? The answers are not always clear.

There are stressors other than these sexual and romantic minefields that should be mentioned. Out on the floors, women physicians sometimes find they are subject to competency judgments by their patients, hospital support personnel, and colleagues. On occasion, patients, male and female, assume, sometimes rather vocally, that all female medical personnel must be nurses. When instructed otherwise, the patients may inquire if a "real doctor" is also involved in their care.

Sometimes supporting coworkers may also harbor inherent value judgments about the relative competency of male and female physicians. Studies have demonstrated, for example, female physicians often feel that they receive less respect and displays of confidence from their nursing colleagues than do their male counterparts.[3] This sort of attitude may be reinforced by certain male physicians' more boisterous and more assertive take-control behaviors when interacting with patients and medical teammates. People often believe what they are more assertively told. Yet, female physician assertiveness often seems to be greeted with far less respect, warmth, and compliance.

We have noted elsewhere in this book that women must deal, more directly at least, with the decisions and ramifications related to pregnancy and child rearing. They are thus often subjected to the tug of war between home and career. They are not alone, but somehow men have been given more of a societal and professional "bye" here. In this era of dual-career parenting, studies have demonstrated that men have been remarkably remiss in picking up an equal share of related responsibilities.

There is a not-so-subtle professional toll to this dynamic. When at home, women are more likely to attend to family needs, whereas men are more likely to engage in work-related activities such as preparing grants and writing academic papers. Women's professional productivity and advancement could run the risk of lagging until their families have matured.[4]

Furthermore, with men filling most medical leadership positions, women have potentially fewer role models to emulate and mentors to help usher them into various professional "fast tracks."

The sum total of many of these factors leads to an inherent industry bias against the advancement of women to the highest positions of leadership—a further stress for those who aspire to such professional levels.

Here are a few questions for you to contemplate and discuss with your peers, friends, families, mentors, or perhaps a therapist. Please see www.studergroup.com/thriving-physician for more questions.

Consider and Discuss

- What are your own perceptions of female physicians? How do they differ from male physicians? Who would you prefer caring for you? Why? What about physicians of different ethnicities, political persuasions, sexual orientation, religion?

- How often do you witness sexism, misogyny, or over-sexualized comments or behaviors in your workplace? What do you do about it? What should/can you do about it?

- Are hyper-flexible work schedules possible in medicine? How about part-time positions? How should these schedules affect professional standing and advancement? How about reimbursement?

- How should an institution codify and handle romantic/sexual interaction between coworkers? Should workplaces have zero-tolerance policies on fraternization between coworkers? What are the possible negative consequences of such policies?

- How can we make the workplace more hospitable for women? For minorities? For people of other diverse cultures and backgrounds?

Building Resilience

If you are a female physician, know that we are at the dawn of a much brighter era in medicine. Some of the needed changes are coming, and they are probably accelerating due to overall cultural evolution within our society. Nonetheless, sexual harassment still occurs and should be considered unacceptable. Let's not mince words here. Sexual harassment is a heinous act. It is an aggressive and threatening behavior. It diminishes you as a person and degrades your effectiveness as a physician.

- Don't face harassment alone. Most medical systems have active human resources programs and internal legal departments to help you deal with egregious behaviors, and you should avail yourself of these and any other available resources. If you bring issues to these entities, insist that they do their jobs. Put the onus on them and be willing to press the issue. If the offender is in your direct chain of command, you will feel intimidated to take action, but it is imperative not to let offensive or aggressive behaviors take root. Enlist your colleagues, male and female, around you. If the behaviors are overt, there will be others who have witnessed them or have suffered through them themselves.

- Be aware that some well-meaning people don't realize that their dialogue or behaviors are offensive, demeaning, or threatening. You can do your part by addressing such issues upfront and by educating. It does not have to be confrontational, and any person worth their salt will take such correction to heart. By addressing such issues directly, you will gain back some sense of control and empowerment. The behaviors will hopefully diminish (perhaps not without repeated reminders), and the workplace may become more enjoyable again.

- Sexualized dialogue or behavior, racial slurs, or demeaning language should not be tolerated even from your patients. Gently correct misbehaving patients by addressing their behaviors directly and explaining why they are offensive and unacceptable. It is okay to terminate a professional relationship with a patient if they are persistently abusive. Involve your patient representative office if need be.

- As a physician, male or female, turn your radar on to your own behavior and that of those around you. Shaping a respectful and tolerant workplace culture requires unrelenting, mindful collaboration between all workers. Remember, there are many about you who are vulnerable. There are many who are susceptible to slight or inappropriate behavior. There are many who have not enjoyed even a modicum of power or privilege or social approbation.

- Consider the plight of members of the various races, sexual orientations, religions, and cultures around you. Before any demeaning commentary of any kind ever leaves your lips, bite your tongue and hold it in. Think about the corrosive effects such comments may have. Recognize that no joke that diminishes the worth of another being, no matter how funny it may seem to you, is worth the potential negative effects it has on those around you.

- Create a warm, welcoming, supportive environment for all people around you. Be a safe haven for all your coworkers. Notice bad behaviors about you and address them. And please, approach the victim and demonstrate to him or her that he or she is not responsible, and that he or she does not have to face it alone.

- Take it upon yourself to help change the culture within your institution, not just for women but for all. Treat all as equals. Acknowledge each other's accomplishments and qualities as people and professionals. Honor diversity. Show compassion for each other's work/life dynamics and the strains they may create. The more the hospitable and nurturing your work environment for all, the greater will be your own enjoyment and personal development.

- Become aware of the power differentials that exist in almost all professional relationships and how you personally, or others, may use or tacitly benefit from them.

- Think about how you can mentor those below you and help advance their careers—particularly those from groups who traditionally have not enjoyed such advancement in your field. Celebrate their successes.

CHAPTER THIRTEEN

A Billion Here, a Billion There, and Pretty Soon You're Talking About Real Money

—Widely attributed to Everett M. Dirksen

The Persistent Stress of Debt

"The lack of money is the root of all evil."

—Mark Twain

George Bailey: *I know one way you can help me. You don't happen to have 8,000 bucks on you?*

Clarence: *No, we don't use money in Heaven.*

George Bailey: *Well, it comes in real handy down here, bud!*

—It's a Wonderful Life

Few members of the general public are moved to much pity for the financially "struggling" doctor. But the truth is that most physicians in training and in early practice are actually rather poor. Most have absorbed debt from the incomprehensible $280,000 (or more) cost of four years at medical school (on average) and their undergraduate education costs. Then, resident salaries, although significantly improved from days gone by, are still far from lavish (average $55,000 per year in 2018—for 80 hours of work a week!).

> *On surveying residents across the country, their scholastic debt ranged from $300,000 to $700,000 (from pre-medical and medical school tuition and living expenses). While they kept up with their interest payments, most noted that it was nearly impossible to make inroads on their principals. Some felt it was not even worth trying during training, incurring substantially further debt to affect an enjoyable standard of living.*

Most residents add to their debt throughout training, deferring the pain of repayment to a time when they hopefully will be earning a "real salary." But debts in the several hundred thousand dollars take a long time to pay off. Many residents believe that they will negotiate debt repayment upfront when they sign up for their first job, but this is not a given in the modern medical universe.

If you are in training or in early practice, you may soothe your financial worries by believing that at some point down the line you will realize a very comfortable living. And for most physicians, this is the case. But the time it takes to reach financial solvency may be many years, even decades. Financial stress and worry will likely be a part of your life for quite some time.

If you are like most, you worry about both current and future finances. You worry whether you will eventually find a reasonable job, or whether your current job will be remunerative enough to start making it to the positive side of the ledger. You worry about the future of medical economics in the country. You worry about becoming disabled enough, through injury or illness, that you might not be able to someday realize a truly healthy salary.

What is more, financial splurging is a common response to the severe self-denial and delayed gratification that the profession demands. Many residents and physicians describe an irresistible urge to buy. Buy what? Things—meaningless and extravagant objects of temporary desire, with no real value to the purchaser. These purchases may not even fit into a hobby or personal interest of the purchaser. They are bought out of compulsion. Often, purchased items go completely unused.

Others will head to the casinos or take part in other overly expensive activities. It seems that the act of spending serves as a release of self-denial tension and/or as a perceived "pay-back" to loved ones who have suffered the physicians' long periods of work-related absence. But it is an empty and generally very temporary release. Thus, a new cycle of purchasing is certain to follow. Spendthrift behavior in the face of severe debt heightens personal tension, fuels guilt, perpetuates financial anxiety, and may severely strain relationships with significant others.

Here are a few questions for you to contemplate and discuss with your peers, friends, families, mentors, or perhaps a therapist. Please see www.studergroup.com/thriving-physician for more questions.

Consider and Discuss

- Do you financially splurge when "released" from work? On what? What pleasure does it bring you? What financial impact does this have?

- What type of lifestyle is important to you? What material goods do you crave? When you climb out of the financial hole, how will your lifestyle change?

- What purchases do you own that you seldom or never use?

- Have you received any financial counseling? Have you read any books on personal finance? What were the key lessons/recommendations?

- How many others depend on your financial solvency?

- Do you think about retirement? At what age do you think you will retire? What will you do with yourself when you do retire? How long will it take to be financially able to retire?

Building Resilience

Unless you are really lucky, you will face (and are likely already facing) profound financial concerns. It is critical to accept that this anxiety will be a part of your life for quite some time. Be mindful of its impact on you and your loved ones. Seek to be frugal to lessen its impact. For example:

- Look for outlets from self-denial other than shopping/spending/financial extravagance. Activities like hiking, gardening, reading, or just hanging out with friends are cheap or free and can be remarkably rewarding.

- Seek *experiences* over material goods.
- Remember: Spending begets spending. It becomes a habit or a personal culture that is difficult to break away from. Living simply and frugally can also be made into a personal culture. The more this is practiced, the easier it is to do.
- Read personal finance books. Seek financial counseling.
- Be open about your state of finances and your financial concerns with your loved ones. Share fiscal responsibility—don't go it alone.
- Establish a pattern of saving, even if the amounts are minimal. Take pride in money saved rather than spent.
- Chip away at debt. Don't let it grow by a slow unnoticeable creep. Do the opposite by attacking it in small bites all the time. Even small increments will reduce anxiety to some degree. The impact on your lifestyle will not be perceptible but the impact year to year can be profound.
- Keep a definitive ledger of your expenses and review it periodically. Ask yourself if the money spent makes sense.
- Remember that "financial resilience," just like general resilience, is made up of small choices, each of which may seem inconsequential in the moment.

CHAPTER FOURTEEN

Garbage in, Garbage Out

Information Overload

"Man's mind, once stretched by a new idea, never regains its original dimensions."
—*Oliver Wendell Holmes*

"I don't think much of a man who is not wiser today than he was yesterday."
—*Abraham Lincoln*

On a regular basis, you likely leave your exhausting day of work only to submerge yourself into the textbooks and professional journals of your specialty that evening. If you are a resident, the specters of attending rounds, grand rounds, "pimping sessions," in-service exams, written boards, and oral boards are ever-present. And so you dig further into the scientific underpinnings of your chosen discipline: anatomy, physiology, radiology, pathology, pathophysiology, pharmacology, and the like. If you are a practicing physician, you likely have realized that your learning curve will never level off. The advances in your specialty are endless, and there will always be the specter of recertification and the need for amassing continuing education credits looming…for your entire career.

Being a physician requires you to tackle a vast volume of knowledge. The study of physiology alone, in any single organ system, could be a life's work. And consider pharmacology—can anyone keep up with all the new medications out there? The task feels insurmountable.

Specialists must digest every intricate nuance of their fields. Meanwhile, those in primary or frontline care must learn about…well…everything!

Regardless of your career stage, you can add mastering all the information and knowledge behind your chosen discipline of medicine to your list of tasks that will never be completely accomplished. This fact may make you anxious, particularly if you are perfectionistic (and most of you out there are!).

A particularly painful part of the psychology of residency (and medicine in general) is that performance anxiety compounds itself daily as you are surrounded by people who know more about your specialty than you do. Historically, one of the principal methodologies of medical training revolved around the open demonstration of precisely what you did *not* know. (Think of rounds, and "pimping," and the Socratic method.) The methodology still has its advocates (G. Simonds for one!). With all of the distractions of modern-day multi-media life, a degree of embarrassment is a strong driver of scholarly behavior. But it comes at the cost of increased anxiety about what is not known.

The need for "more home study" will be a constant threat to your resilience-restoring personal time. You will need to learn to manage a resilience double-bind here: You should create more time for yourself and your well-being. Yet, daily you may be shamed (by others or yourself) for not knowing every intricacy of a disorder and its management. Guilt and anxiety will creep in, particularly when you try to enjoy restorative activities. It will also show up when you get caught in a profound knowledge gap on rounds, or when a patient does poorly and you feel that you missed something in their diagnosis or care.

> *On surveying residents across the country, the grand majority reported significant unease at taking prolonged breaks from their studies. They noted that guilt occurred when they went more than an hour at home without studying. Most found that they simply could not take an entire day off, no matter what.*

It does not get much easier after training, particularly during the early years of a medical career. Young physicians are besieged with feelings and fears of inadequacy regarding their clinical competence. They often feel like an imposter: "I can't really care for this patient; I don't know anything!" They realize that they cannot know everything, but now they are responsible for the safety and health of their patients.

The remedy is to read more, study more, and learn more. Many young physicians report reading more in the first five years of practice than they did during their residencies. Many report running to handbooks and web resources every time they evaluate a new patient.

This raises the question: Can you ever stop the incessant studying? Unlikely. Even if you are a seasoned physician in practice, you must review and rehearse already-learned medical knowledge throughout your career and constantly incorporate new knowledge. In fact, most specialties require periodic passing of "maintenance of competency" exams. A whole industry of related educational resources has exploded in response. Adding fuel to the fire, the hallowed halls of academic medicine drive "scholarly works" factories via their publish-or-perish cultures—bombarding you with their product (useful or not).

The scope of modern medical knowledge is mind-blowing and ever-expanding. The array of journals, websites, seminars, scientific meetings, courses, and webinars available to modern physicians is stupefying. No one can attend to it all let alone incorporate it all. It's a perfectionist's nightmare!

> *Practicing physicians interviewed reported to us significant "journal pile guilt." That is, their guilt levels rose proportional to the height of the pile of unread professional journals within their homes. Several reported difficulty being in the same room as the pile, once it reached a certain height. Others reported throwing a blanket over the pile so it could not shame them!*

This is the learning challenge you face throughout your career. It is up to you to filter it all with a critical eye and separate out the medical wheat from the chaff. And then study it, understand it, remember it, and incorporate it into your practice. Good luck with that!

If you're a Millennial, you may believe you have the solution. After all, you grew up in the information era. You have the world's accumulated knowledge at your fingertips. So why bother pounding all this stuff into your heads when you can quickly look it up online? Doesn't all that forced learning and memorization interfere with your creativity and originality?

Here is the rub. Modern cognitive science is beginning to discover that total dependence on IT and perhaps AI may be detrimental to your processing. It appears that if you do not memorize things, you won't remember them or their context, and you may be less able to process conceptualizations about them.[1]

In other words, by failing to learn and memorize new information, we may be atrophying our cognitive powers rather than facilitating further creativity. Think about it. How easy is it to mentally manipulate a complex concept if you have little or no understanding of its fundamentals? Furthermore, we are constantly awash in information. How can you choose which information to process and manipulate if *all* information appears of equivalent value because it does not resonate with stored knowledge in your brain? Just some food for thought.

Here are a few questions for you to contemplate and discuss with your peers, friends, families, mentors, or perhaps a therapist. Please see www.studergroup.com/thriving-physician for more questions.

Consider and Discuss

- When was the first time you encountered the quandary of caring deeply about something, committing to being excellent in that endeavor, and realizing that, no matter how hard you worked at it, you would never fully master it?

- In any endeavor, how did you then decide what was a "good enough" effort on your part?

- If perfection in medicine is not possible, how do you reconcile your level of expertise with the notion of perfection?

- How can you make lifelong learning enjoyable and efficient?

- What environment do you need to accomplish effective and efficient studying? How easy is it to establish said environment in your current life?

Building Resilience

When it comes to building an academic knowledge base, perfectionism can truly hold you back. You simply cannot read it all, address it all, learn it all, understand it all, and incorporate it all. This is a compromise you have to make in medicine—to set a limit on how much you will digest day to day, year to year. But this should not be an excuse not to stay current in your discipline.

Instead, periodically put some real thought into your approach to learning, rather than allowing yourself to be overwhelmed by the tidal wave of materials coming at you.

- Sit down and map out your study plans.
- Schedule your study time over weeks and months. Write it down.
- Note which educational materials and methods work best for you. Make sure you have access to these resources.
- Don't try to keep up with dozens of journals and websites. Select those that are the most interesting, relevant, and efficacious for you.
- Create a routine that supports maximum efficacy and efficiency.
- Incorporate your study schedule into your "wellness schedule." Make sure there is time for both.
- Assess periodically how the "dance" between the two is going. Do you feel too guilty and anxious about lack of studying, or too burned out by lack of time for yourself and loved ones? Adjust accordingly.
- Remember: You will drift to inertia unless you put energy into changing things for the better.
- Consider arranging your educational activities in boluses. Go to national meetings or courses. Perhaps schedule a block of journal reading Sunday afternoon once a month.
- Employ multi-media learning. Download audible materials for time in the car. Check out specialty-related apps for your phone.
- Host a journal club. What better way to couple lifelong learning with fellowship and camaraderie (build the team as you build your mind).

CHAPTER FIFTEEN

On a Runaway Train

Lack of Control

"You must learn to let go. Release the stress. You were never in control anyway."
—*Steve Maraboli*

"You may not control all the events that happen to you, but you can decide not to be reduced by them."
—*Maya Angelou*

Work settings characterized by *high demand, low control* (over your work flow and decision latitude), and low interpersonal and/or institutional *support*, are toxic cauldrons that breed burnout and many other maladaptive responses. Such work settings have been shown to be dangerous to your health.[1]

A critical component is lack of control. It does not matter whether this is perceived or actual. In the face of challenges and demands, the absence of decision latitude—the ability to decide what is to be done and how to do it—is poisonous, particularly for high performers. Resilience is far more susceptible to a sense of lack of control than it is to extreme hard work. When your sense of control is compromised, defensive shields come down, and burnout easily ensues.

All physicians certainly deal with a growing lack of control in the modern medical world. So much of the autonomy, authority, and independence enjoyed in the "gilded age" has been ceded to other entities. Think of the challenges provided by the vagaries of today's large healthcare systems and their requisite bureaucracies. They oft reach Orwellian proportions.

> *Our department was recently informed that it was losing hundreds of thousands of dollars "for the system" because of the way it was requesting in-patient imaging studies. Without certain "key words" and phrases in the requests, payments for the images were being denied. The administrators bearing the news, however, could not provide the requisite key words that would obviate the problem—just the terms that did not work. Nonetheless, compliance with using the proper terminology was made part of our physicians' "scorecards," potentially threatening a portion of their pay. The team was thus being penalized for lack of compliance with mandates that were not, and could not, be defined. Kafka could not come up with something better than this!*

If you are like most other physicians, you more and more feel that you have very limited control over your high-demand life. Your work is overseen by senior physicians, hospital administrators, nursing supervisors, hospital committees, healthcare organizations, insurance companies, specialty governing bodies, the state and federal governments, and more. If you run afoul of any of these entities, you may have to address formal complaints or rebukes; you may even find yourself before an official board or government investigator.

If you are a resident, you get it in spades. You are asked to accept a life of servitude. Hierarchy is the way of life, and you are at the bottom. Every thought, decision, action, intervention you enact must be approved, and then is subject to dissection, correction, and critique. Many see residency as entailing a total surrender of autonomy, independence, and authority. For some, this state of existence persists for seven or more years. You thus face the "perfect burnout storm" of extremely hard work, excessive hours, and essentially no control over your current condition.

In addition, the practice of clinical medicine does not lend itself to superlative control. Stuff happens, often unexpectedly. Even when expected, it often cannot be controlled. And, when things "go south," they often seem to snowball toward total disaster. One little event begets a bigger one, and so forth. Thus, you feel driven to control even the smallest of circumstances, believing you may be heading off larger disasters down the line. We have all experienced the hyper-attentive clinician who must know every trivial detail about every patient in his or her care. Control freak? Micromanager? Or just someone trying to keep his or her head "above water"?

Here are a few questions for you to contemplate and discuss with your peers, friends, families, mentors, or perhaps a therapist. Please see www.studergroup.com/thriving-physician for more questions.

Consider and Discuss

- Are there opportunities in the course of your daily work for you to exercise control over what you do or how you go about doing it? How about at home?
- Is it possible that you have more control over your environment than you believe? In what ways?
- Are there any advantages to surrendering control (e.g., lack of responsibility or culpability)?
- Who truly has a large amount of control over their lives? Is it real control or perceived? How do they respond to this?

Building Resilience

As noted in the quotations that started this chapter, control over anything in life is a rather elusive, ephemeral, and probably fallacious concept. It can be particularly tough to develop resilience in this area. Giving up a burning need to maintain control of all that goes on about you would be a great start. You know, relax, chill, "don't sweat the small stuff."

It's a great philosophy, but it is far easier said than done; and it certainly doesn't help you manage a 50-patient medical service. Still, a modicum of the right "philosophy" can help soothe excessive need for control and can go a very long way to help sustain resilience. This is known as deploying a "default philosophy." It can help steer your thinking patterns, and these thinking patterns can have positive emotional and behavioral consequences. In other words, sometimes it is of great benefit to deliberately direct your conscience to positive thoughts (even clichés) in troublesome and stressful times. In this case: "Chill, don't sweat the small stuff."

Also keep in mind that you have more control than you realize. If you are a resident, consider this: Although it is an exercise in delayed gratification, you are preparing for a long, gratifying career in medicine that virtually guarantees a steady income and societal respect and gratitude. By your hard work and focus, and even your surrendering of some control now, you are controlling your future. There is something to be said about that! Don't be afraid to remind yourself what it is all about. Always keep in mind a positive vision of your future.

- If you are a resident, enjoy the rare privilege of controlling your own destiny. If you are a practicing physician, you are there! Revel in it!

- Remember that you maintain near total control of who you are and how you present yourself to the outside world. Although you may develop "blurry vision" about this when you are extraordinarily stressed, it's still true. If you are a warm, smiling, loving, and caring person, it is because you have chosen to be so. If you work to sustain this, you will be treated better, you will feel better, and you will be afforded more opportunities to control other aspects of your life.

- If you are in a supervisory position over residents and/or other physicians (and/or support personnel), seek to enable their sense of control. Simple measures may go a long way toward lessening the high demand/low control dynamic. Research with health professionals has shown that boosting workers' decision latitude significantly counteracts stress and boosts resilience.[2] Some suggestions follow, but many others can and should be generated:
  - Have the residents/support personnel/junior physicians make their own call and vacation schedules.
  - Don't set hard-and-fast rules on time off. Let those under you set the limits. (They may surprise you by being more restrictive on themselves and each other than you would be. Most physicians do not want to burden each other with cross-coverage.)
  - Give all team members a full voice, and potentially a representative vote, in the selection of new residents, as well as new advanced care practitioners, attending physicians, and support personnel.
  - Give team members a major role in the planning of the yearly academic schedule, including rotations, subjects, texts, journal clubs, assignments, and improvements.
  - Have team members decide who will go to various courses and national meetings.

- Have the residents decide who will attend the operative cases, procedures, clinics of the day/week.

- Routinely solicit from all team members suggestions on program improvement. Make sure that they see that you act upon at least some of their suggestions.

- Solicit from all team members real feedback on the performance of attending physicians, ACPs, nurses, and support personnel. Make sure they see you act upon their 360 degrees feedback.

- When team members bring you problems or request assistance, ask for their input about how the problem might be addressed. Then make sure they see swift and decisive action from you.

CHAPTER SIXTEEN

Where's the Cavalry?

Lack of Support

"Be strong; be fearless. And believe that anything is possible when you have the right people there to support you."

—*Misty Copeland*

"A man's pride can be his downfall, and he needs to learn when to turn to others for support and guidance."

—*Bear Grylls*

Burnout flourishes in professional settings that rob you of a sense of control *and* a sense of adequate and appropriate support. In fact, one fosters the other. It is hard to "charge up San Juan Hill" if you look over your shoulder and see no one charging with you. Modern medicine is hyper-complex and depends on coordinated teams of professionals assisting the frontline providers. Nowadays, this means non-medical personnel as well as physicians, advanced care practitioners, nurses, and technicians.

Take our world—neurosurgery—for example. The simple act of handing a neurosurgeon an instrument whilst he or she is operating under a microscope can either be a beautiful ballet of synchronized, unspoken thought and movement or a circus act of fumbling frustration.

One of our surgeons tells of a particularly passive-aggressive "scrub tech," who, when disaffected (which was often), would hold instruments a centimeter or two out of the surgeon's comfortable reach. Over and over again.

When teamwork falters, reason would suggest that you could and should openly discuss improvement initiatives with receptive teammates. If a reasonable and direct approach fails, you would expect there to be an approachable support infrastructure and chain of command to which you could express concerns. Ideally, this would include both clinical and administrative leaders who would swiftly correct the problems. Medicine would be far less stressful if such support universally existed. Unfortunately, this chain of support may not materialize. In its absence, you can easily become frustrated, angry, and fearful (for the quality of your care and the safety of your patient).

Given the trials and tribulations of your typical workday, your peace of mind is at profound risk if institutional, functional, and moral support are not available when needed. (And, please, don't get us started on your unavoidable interface with the ubiquitous and omnipotent electronic medical records system and the armies of technological support personnel.) Lack of perceived support regarding issues that trouble you will fuel a sense of lack of control. This combination can leave you floundering in a sea of futility and learned helplessness.

The more complicated, integrated, technical, and high-stakes the medical activity, the more complex the psychosocial challenges, and the more sensitive you become to any perceived lack of assistance. On the other hand, even simple tasks become excruciating without effective teamwork. High performance depends on a network of support through almost every function in a day's work. You are on the very front lines of the delivery of healthcare. The more dysfunctional the support, the more combustible the tinderbox of your frustration, fear, disappointment, and disaffection.

Here are a few questions for you to contemplate and discuss with your peers, friends, families, mentors, or perhaps a therapist. Please see www.studergroup.com/thriving-physician for more questions.

Consider and Discuss

- Think about your various work settings. Which are the units and teams with whom you most enjoy working? Why? What boosts your comfort when working with these teams or units? What characterizes those people and units with whom you least enjoy working? How do *you* behave differently with these two groups of individuals and teams?

- What are measures *you* can initiate that may encourage allied health personnel and administrators to better support your mission? Consider preceding a need/request/fix by these words: "Susan, thank you for all you do for this team…" (gratitude isn't just for the receiver).

- Do you ask for help? Are you annoyed when help is not spontaneously offered? What stories do you tell yourself about people who are not helping or offering help? Do you offer help to non-physicians? Do you offer to help non-medical personnel?

- Do you feel like a part of a functional team, or like a solo player? What makes you feel one way or the other? What would make you feel more part of a team? Do you want to be part of a team?

- How often do you tell your support team that they are doing a great job, that they are valuable members of the team, that they have contributed greatly to the well-being of your patients? How often do you consider their psychological well-being? How can you add to their enjoyment of their work?

- Have you made it easy for administration to focus, fix, and follow up on process breakdowns, tools, and equipment needs? Being solutions-minded and offering that golden lens of clinical clarity goes a long way for the operational leader who wants to help but may not understand your "game."

Building Resilience

The era of the "lone wolf" practitioner is over. Almost by necessity, you will spend much of your professional life working in teams and for systems. You may not always be able to impact the functionality of your system, but you certainly can impact those supporting you every day: your team(s). Realize who makes up your team. Consider how to maximize their functionality with respect to your mission.

Remember two risks that can inadvertently complicate your practice of medicine. The first is totally ignoring members of your team—treating them as role players, not human beings who are affected by what is going on about them, and by your interactions with them. The second is seeing your workplace colleagues as impediments and/or annoyances. This trap may be hard to avoid. Someone has to get you to sign the insurance forms and physical therapy consults. Someone has to report the phone call from an upset patient. Someone has to remind you to watch the system's diversity video, or to close your charts in the EMR. It is so easy to vent your frustrations on the messenger. And of course, they are adding tasks to your already over-taxed day.

Remind yourself that most of these people respect you and some are even intimidated by you. Any sign that you are annoyed with them will likely complicate your relationship. A sarcastic remark or a barking rebuke can be devastating. But even your subtlest change in demeanor will likely be noticed. And you may actually employ this not too subtly with non-verbal language that says, "Go away; leave me alone!" It can be difficult to shut down this response. Remind yourself that staff are not paid to be your punching bag, and they surely did not sign up to share your frustrations about your institution, the electronic medical record, or about the entire American healthcare system.

- Notice who your team members are. Learn their names. You are so busy that these very real human beings can become a piece of the scenery. Stopping for a moment, making eye contact with them, and showing pleasure at their presence takes milliseconds. People are far more likely to assist you if they like you and respect you, and we all tend to like and respect people who seem to care about us.
- Know a little bit about your teammates—the real them, not their hospital personae. Inquire periodically about their families and activities.
- Remember, you are not the only one in the healthcare universe who is at high risk for burnout. The nurses, physician assistants, technicians, and other healthcare personnel are very much feeling the strain as well.
- Show genuine concern for teammates who are sick or exhibit distress.
- Offer to help teammates with their duties.
- Notice your teammates' efforts. Compliment them. Thank them. There's no need to be cloying or insincere, but a little effort on your part can pay off in spades.

- Brag about the efforts of your team and specific teammates to the chain of command. "Write up" efforts that were above and beyond the call of duty or that were particularly creative or inspired.
- Share credit for accomplishments with your whole team.
- Educate your team on what exactly you are trying to do for your patients. Teach them about the disorders they will interface with. Show them stellar results. Introduce them to happy patients.
- Consider constructing a simple reward system for excellence in your teammates' efforts; perhaps coffee shop gift cards or certificates of appreciation, etc.
- Work on team spirit. Consider identifying apparel such as baseball caps or t-shirts.
- Consider hosting "retreats" with your team featuring picnics, lunches, bowling, etc.
- Always speak in terms of "we" rather than "I" when discussing the care of your patients.
- Forgive mistakes. Educate your teammates rather than rant or admonish.
- Smile a lot at your teammates. Make them feel you are genuinely happy to see them and interact with them.
- Listen intently to the suggestions of your teammates. You may be surprised at how smart, observant, and contributory they can be.

Regarding Your Overall System:

- Get to know your administrators. Talk to them, socialize a bit with them, understand their constraints. If you are a physician leader (chair, chief, division head, or medical director), consider quarterly "rounding on the C-suite" to ensure you and they are aligned on shared goals and aware of issues in the workplace. Thirty minutes of this type of collegial interaction will save hours of frustration and create a team environment from top to bottom.
- Reason with, don't rant at, your administrative chain of command. They are far more likely to seek to help you if they like and respect you.
- Realize that many constraints are beyond anyone's control. Healthcare is a bureaucratic behemoth with byzantine governmental rules and guidelines that may make affecting certain changes next to impossible. Learn to work within these constraints and focus your energies on things you can improve.
- Show up! Make it to hospital committee meetings, departmental meetings, medical center meetings, and the like. You cannot influence positive change anonymously. Be an engaged listener and voice.

CHAPTER SEVENTEEN

Decisions, Decisions, Decisions

Relentless Decision-Making

"The most difficult thing is the decision to act; the rest is merely tenacity."

—Amelia Earhart

"In any moment of decision, the best thing you can do is the right thing, the next best thing is the wrong thing, and the worst thing you can do is nothing."

—Theodore Roosevelt

"Sometimes you make the right decision; sometimes you make the decision right."

—Phil McGraw

You are called upon to make decisions, great and small, every couple of minutes, throughout each working day. The bigger, more complex, and more important decisions are somehow easier to take—they are what all your years of training were about. It is the little niggling ones that are irksome, and they seem to come at you relentlessly. It is the way of modern medicine. It is the case in the clinic setting, the emergency room, the operating room, and even within the hospital. There, nursing responsibility for on-the-spot patient decision making seems to have been reduced to near comic lows. This is ironic considering the push for greater and greater nursing autonomy, and the sky-high admission criteria for entry into nursing school.

It feels as if nurses are no longer entrusted with even the most rudimentary patient care decisions. Thus, frontline physicians are routinely called to grant nurses permission to execute the most pedantic of tasks: catheterize a patient with a bladder residual urine volume of 1000cc, give a laxative to a patient who has not had a bowel movement for five days, change the soiled dressings of a surgical wound.

There was a time when such decisions were made on the floor by a patient's nurse and simply documented in the patient's chart or relayed to the provider team the next day on rounds. No longer! You are flooded with these calls night and day. Mixed in are critical inquiries on ICU patients, immediate post-operative patients, emergency room patients, and patients exhibiting major changes in their conditions. The net effect is a near constant and perpetual bombardment of calls necessitating rapid adjudication of patient care issues ranging from the farcical to the hyper-emergent, and everything in between.

Of course, this carries some problematic fallout. Firstly, the activity is exhausting. Your mind is granted no time to contemplate the problems presented; you just react and solve. Before you have time to ponder your previous decision, the next wave of questions and requests arrives. You often get to enjoy 12 straight hours of this; if on-call, 24 to 36 hours of it.

> *Periodically, our physician assistants take the primary "pager" for our residents for a few hours. These battle-hardened warriors report being absolutely drained by the end of such an activity. They feel overwhelmed and battered. They report that the weight of the near-constant decision-making is simply oppressive. They note that it takes hours to fully recover from the experience.*

Sometimes, your shifts fill with the constant drone of low-level decision-making. You wonder whether your years of training and hundreds of thousands of dollars of schooling truly culminate solely in your competency as a bowel movement manager. Time is such a critical factor in your life. Yet it feels so squandered after hours of fielding "inconsequential" requests and inquiries.

You may find it difficult to shut off the problem-solving mindset. At home, you will encounter loved ones who simply want to chat about the trials and tribulations of their days—big and small. Often, they just want a sympathetic ear. You, however, will kick into problem-solving mode and immediately start to decree solutions: "Billy did not want to do his homework to-night" therefore *"okay, no video games for a week."* "The car battery indicator light is still on after it was in the shop all week" therefore *"okay, demand our money back and take it to another shop."* The solutions are not thought-out in depth, or with all contexts and outcomes weighed with insight and wisdom. Rather, they are exercises in expediency and efficiency.

Your loved ones will find such behavior tiresome if not outright irksome. Seldom do they feel unequipped to handle their own daily issues or those of their families. In fact, they find it insulting and belittling when their chatter about the day is greeted with an uncontestable edict from the "Lord (or Lady)-high-almighty of the house."

Here are a few questions for you to contemplate and discuss with your peers, friends, families, mentors, or perhaps a therapist. Please see www.studergroup.com/thriving-physician for more questions.

Consider and Discuss

- How can you control your negative emotions and responses to trivial questions?
- How can you validate the person making calls to you?
- Would you support more nursing autonomy? What should be the limits? Who should decide? To what degree should you be responsible if mistakes are made?
- How often do you bring your "court of last appeal" persona home? How do others respond to it? How might you modify it?
- Is that "trivial" concern or request of your patient all that trivial to your patient?

Building Resilience

Like so many of the challenges you face, this one isn't going away any time soon. And so, you are going to have to learn to deal with it constructively. Every call is an opportunity to color another person's perception of you. You can rapidly build a network of friends and admirers, or you can construct a cavalcade of people who don't think all that highly of you. Which option will work better for your functionality within the hospital? Which will make you feel better?

Yes, a momentary burst of sarcasm or worse can relieve the tension of your frustration, but in the long run, it will erode your happiness. Most people don't fare well as the proverbial ogre. It feels much better to be nice to others and to be liked. So when called:

- Pick up the phone, smile, and pleasantly attend to what is asked of you.
- When a pleasant demeanor is not easily forthcoming for you, force a smile onto your countenance. You will be surprised at how it changes your intonation.
- When a nurse's first line begins with "Dr. Smith, sorry to bother you, but the patient in Room 232…" preface your answer with: "You are not a bother and thanks for inquiring about…"
- Tack on a sincere "thank you" and "have a great day" to all your phone conversations.
- Consider the lot of the person on the other end of the call. Did they really set out today to annoy you, or are they trying to do their job as prescribed by others? Are they truly concerned about one of *your* patients? Do they need direction or affirmation? Are they young and inexperienced? Are they frightened by what is going on before them? Treat someone who is truly nervous or in need well, and you have an ally for life.
- Remember the lot of the patient. They are strangers in a strange land. What seems like a trivial issue to you may feel monumental to them. An infiltrated IV may be an everyday event to you, but to them it is a frightening and very uncomfortable phenomena. When a nurse asks for your assistance or guidance with a patient, do your best to focus on the discomfort of the patient and seek to alleviate it.
- When you get home, put the judge's wig and robe away. Give yourself and your loved ones a break from your decision-making persona and simply listen. Escape your world and live on the outside for a while through theirs. Offer empathy and affirmation. If they want decision-making support or wise solutions, they will ask for it.

CHAPTER EIGHTEEN

Am I Really a Doctor or Am I a Poser?

Ego Battering

"There is overwhelming evidence that the higher the level of self-esteem, the more likely one will be to treat others with respect, kindness, and generosity."

—Nathaniel Branden

"Self-love, my liege, is not so vile a sin, as self-neglecting."

—William Shakespeare

Surprisingly, physicians often suffer from severely ailing egos. This is ironic because a fairly strong ego is needed to care for the sick. The risk-taking and educated guessing involved in patient care demands a certain level of self-confidence and trust in one's own judgment. You have to believe that you can competently care for the sick despite the myriad of things that can go wrong.

Granted, most of us come into the profession fairly full of ourselves: straight-A students our entire lives, top of our high school classes, stellar performers in college, cruising through medical school. Few are without a healthy dose of narcissism. But then, the beatings begin.

If you are like most of us, each year of training was a quantum leap in accumulated knowledge, clinical savvy, and technical skill, such that whenever you looked ahead you were reminded how insufficiently developed you were. If you didn't "get it," you were dutifully reminded by your seniors and your attendings, who were all too delighted to probe your medical fiber until its deficiencies were apparent to all (thank you Socrates!). As you approached your chief year, the specter of all the responsibility and decision-making and its attendant self-doubt came flooding in.

And, lest you think the blessed ego salve comes in the attending years, think again. Medicine is a field of strikingly frequent unexpected and poor outcomes. After all, people die. Prior to this, there is a lifetime of slow decline. As a physician, you try to help your patients climb up the "down escalator." But just as you string together a series of happy results, an unexpected and sometimes devastating complication occurs. Many physicians attest that when the "medicine gods" sense that one is down, they pile on an avalanche of other disasters. Just watch the seasoned physician cringe when a simple complication occurs in a cherished patient, as they anxiously wait for the next "boot to drop."

Parenthetically, the seasoned physicians often do not particularly enjoy strings of good results either. Too often in the past, they had allowed themselves to feel good about a procedure or treatment outcome, only to have it crumble before their eyes. Most are therefore too superstitious to truly celebrate any "fruits of their labor" for fear again of inciting the "medicine gods." These are lessons usually learned in residency and never forgotten.

> *One of our medical colleagues recalls an incident early in his training that underscores the point. A young patient underwent a particularly involved intervention with him. Things initially went quite well. Everyone was delighted. The patient's mother baked our colleague a huge pan of delicious fudge in gratitude. Then, a series of devastating complications occurred, one after another. The patient never fully recovered. To this day, our colleague recoils at the mention of fudge, or any baked goods, offered up by a grateful patient or family member.*

Obviously, the assault on your ego will vary with the specialty you have chosen. We in neurosurgery are absolutely pummeled with complications and bad outcomes in our patients. Valiant efforts to manage a tough diabetic in primary care can be crushed by yet another disease complication or unfavorable A1C. But no matter your calling, you want the best for your patients, and results will very often fall short of "the best." So you will have your own wounds to tend to.

> *You might think the diagnostic radiologist is somewhat immune from this. But at least in our program, we make it a point to routinely bring surgical feedback to our neuroradiologists and reference their preoperative interpretations of patient images. Sometimes, the radiologists were unequivocally wrong in their interpretations. And, of course, we are far more likely to bring back negative feedback than positive. So even the radiologists, far removed from actual patient interaction and intervention, are not shielded from the ego battering.*

Also lurking out there is another destroyer of physician egos: litigation. Don't ever believe that you can easily weather a medical lawsuit. It is a savage all-out assault on you and your ego. If you are unlucky enough to be named in a suit, expect to be violated. The plaintiff team will do everything in their power to portray you as uncaring, incompetent, lazy, unprofessional, and unfit to practice. It is a rare individual whose ego can completely withstand this assault. Many physicians never recover from it. We'll talk more about this particular coping challenge later.

Here are a few questions for you to contemplate and discuss with your peers, friends, families, mentors, or perhaps a therapist. Please see www.studergroup.com/thriving-physician for more questions.

Consider and Discuss

- How has your experience in medicine changed your opinion of yourself? Are you able to forgive yourself for your failures and shortcomings?

- Who is capable of helping you when your ego is battered?

- How important is a sound ego in practicing medicine? In caring for the critically ill? In making critical medical decisions? In performing invasive procedures or dangerous medical interventions?

- Where does self-confidence end and over-confidence begin? What type of ego do you want to project to your patients? Your coworkers?

- Who around you seem to have the "right" balance of ego and self-confidence? What is their secret? Can you ask them how they manage complications, bad outcomes, surprises, failures, near-misses, etc.?

Building Resilience

Clearly a healthy ego is critical to efficacy as a physician. If you cannot deflect many of all the insults that medicine can offer up, your ego will suffer and so will your confidence. Your ability to make tough decisions and take calculated risks will be compromised. Thus, recognize that your belief in yourself needs repeated reassessment and often repair.

- Be honest with yourself. This is critical to resilience. Be aware of and track your outcomes.

- Address poor outcomes with thoughtfulness and investigation. Cut yourself some slack, though, particularly after a string of them. You are well trained and well schooled. Chances are these are statistical aberrations—not a condemnation of your overall capabilities. You have to be very careful of anecdotal "confirmation" of your "incompetence" (as well as of your clinical brilliance!). A couple of cases in one direction or the other do not constitute a pattern.

- Seek some form of benchmarking. Ideally, you would track your outcomes and be able to compare them with national norms. If you are within the norms, you can take this as affirmation. If you are way off, it may not indicate a shortcoming, but it should set off warning bells, and it does warrant some investigation of yourself, your approach, your execution, and your institution. If you seem to be under-performing, check off with colleagues, consider refresher courses, read up on the areas in which you seem to be lagging. Be open to coaching and feedback, both key mechanisms for driving performance improvement. (Professional athletes receive both—why not you?)

- Pursue excellence, but be very wary of perfection. Remember, perfection in medicine is a myth. If you insist upon it, you will wear down your ego as well as all your coping mechanisms.

- Make medical self-improvement a central goal to your professional existence. Read a lot, discuss case after case with colleagues, study complications extensively, attend courses, make it to your national scientific meetings, grow with your specialty. This will make you an outstanding clinician, but you will never be perfect. Accept it. Get over it.

- Monitor the status of your ego and "keep it within the navigational beacons." Recognize that it is prone to drifting to extremes. A monumental ego will alienate those about you and will place a target on your back. It will negatively affect your referrals. An ego that is bruised and battered, however, will negatively impact your judgment and your efficacy.

- Remember with humility what got you to where you are. You are amongst the best and the brightest, and you are exquisitely trained. People depend on your intelligence and skills. They therefore also depend on your resilience to the siege upon your ego. So invest time and thought on sustaining it.
- Don't lose sight of the numbers: The vast majority of our clinical decision-making and patient outcomes hit the mark and make a difference in the lives of those entrusted to our care. There will always be tough cases and unintended complications, but keep your sights and focus on your positive impact.

CHAPTER NINETEEN

Cowabunga, Dude

The Shock of Lost Youth

"He had gone to that chest in which he stored his youth and found that, like some armour long unworn, it had rusted away."

—*Adrian Tchaikovsky*, Dragonfly Falling

"Zoom! What was that? That was your life, Mate! Oh, that was quick. Do I get another? Sorry, Mate. That's your lot."

—*John Cleese as Basil Fawlty in* Fawlty Towers

As a pre-medical undergraduate, you likely spent more of your college career in libraries and laboratories than in social gatherings. As a medical student, you buried yourself in books, coming up for air only after major batteries of examinations.

If you are still a resident, you are totally sequestered from the outside world for months at a time. And it is not like the minute you break free of the hospital, you can go out and have some much deserved fun. No. When out of the hospital, you are expected to further your expertise in anatomy; physiology; radiology; pharmacology; indications, risks, and benefits of medical and surgical interventions; procedural techniques; and more. In fact, most residents spend between one and three hours reading textbooks and journals every night. They curtail their sleep to gain more hours, and still have little time for aspects of a "normal" lifestyle that rejuvenate and promote broad psychosocial growth. Put another way, you have very little time to be **you**!

If you are a young, middle career, or older physician, you don't fare much better—particularly if you are a young physician trying to establish a practice, a track record, a reputation, and a standing in your local, regional, and national professional organizations. The average physician in practice puts in 60- to 80-hour workweeks. This time does not include keeping up with advances in their fields, attending conferences, attending committee meetings, doing mandatory EMR and quality training, and more.

Remember, you enter the medical field in your healthiest, most energized years of your life, and you don't come out and cruise in a steady-state, mature practice, until you are at an age where most professional athletes are considered to be "over the hill."

You will invariably experience angst over your lost youth. It will be compounded as you witness the lifestyles of your non-medical friends. In stark contrast to your own confining lifestyle, you will hear of and see (through social media) your friends mountain biking in the Rockies, swimming with the manatees in the Florida Keys, hiking the Andes, partying in Vegas, and so forth.

You will wake up one day and not recognize yourself in the mirror. Your hair will be graying. Your belly will be rounder. Scaling a set of stairs that you once bounded up like a gazelle will feel like a final ascent on Everest. You will notice that you have to hold books further away from your face to read the print. If you attempt a weekend warrior game of soccer, you will be sore in muscles you never knew existed. One benefit, though, is it will take only one or two glasses of wine to sustain a sound "buzz." And, to feel hungover the next day.

Medical students and residents will laugh at your ineptitude with the latest technological advances. Your little toddlers will all of a sudden be going out on dates, shunning your advice, dodging your hugs, and laughing at your musical tastes. You will encourage your significant other to go to bed early with you—not to make love, but to sleep. In other words, you will be old—at least compared to the fresh-faced child who entered medical school.

The sense of lost youth is nothing to be trifled with. Many mature physicians churn with resentment and disenchantment over the issue. They fall prey to what psychologists call the false-hope syndrome: underestimating the effort required to achieve a goal and overestimating the benefits that one will come away with once the goal is achieved.[1]

Even if becoming an established physician yields professional fulfillment, status, and a comfortable income, time, youth, good knees, strong arms, and smooth skin will have disappeared—for good. The delayed gratification that is indigenous to medical residency and early practice seldom delivers the rewards in happiness and fulfillment that had been wagered upon.

Awakening to an older you can be a most terrifying and horrifying shock. It can fill you with panic and even rage and tempt you to recapture your youth in the most unhealthy of ways (affairs, drinking, recreational drugs, extravagant buying, gambling, extreme sports, and other high-risk behaviors). You may feel as if you have been swept into a roaring river, hurtling in the opposite direction of what you desire. You struggle to swim upstream, to return to lost ground, but the current against you is unrelenting and all-powerful.

Here are a few questions for you to contemplate and discuss with your peers, friends, families, mentors, or perhaps a therapist. Please see www.studergroup.com/thriving-physician for more questions.

Consider and Discuss

- How difficult is/was your life as a resident or practicing physician compared to how difficult you thought it would be?

- What are you gaining through your experience as a physician in personal growth, emotional maturation, empathy, human understanding, sensitivity, team-orientation, kindness, caring, and interpersonal skills? Is it worth it? Are your "active lifestyle" friends making similar leaps in personal growth?

- Who around you seems to know the "secret" to "living every day" and "stopping to smell the roses" whilst still working hard? Have you discussed this with them? Can you adopt similar habits?

- What truly brings you happiness and joy right now? How can you engage in this more? Are there other experiences that can generate similar levels of happiness and joy? Will these experiences change over time?

- What is it about aging that is abhorrent to you? Is it fair or helpful for you to feel that way?

Building Resilience

Particle physics and relativity aside, we simply cannot turn back time. We are all in a raging river, and it goes in only one direction. So, beware of trying to make up for lost years by compressing experiences, recreating lost adventures, overcompensating, and/or overindulging. Doing so won't bring back the years. And it can truly lead to disastrous consequences like divorce, alienating your children, financial ruin, addiction, serious injury, or jail. Or, less dramatically, it can leave you with sore muscles, a hangover, and empty, disappointed feelings.

Realize that this paradigm is actually universal and inexorably part of the human condition. Everyone around you is in the river. Contemplations of the passage of time and the relentless journey to oblivion have populated mankind's thoughts and writings since the dawn of civilization. If anything, you are a part of the luckiest generation in history. That is, you are a part of a cohort of humans who will live longer than any that preceded. Your lifespan is double what it was not much more than a century ago. Perhaps, you should be celebrating that the current in the river of life is not as swift as it was for our ancestors.

Of course, this does not solve the problem of cashing in your youth for this career. So, what to do?

- Channel your energies to "living every day."
- Recognize your day-to-day work regimen **is your life.** It needs to be savored and appreciated for what it is—despite the routine and the setting.
- Savor the bursts of humanity, wonder, connection, mystery, magic, craziness, miracle, joy, laughter, community, friendship, and love of the day-to-day. Seek them out, make them happen, share the experience, and revel in it.
- Don't be a zombie. Don't walk through your days in a haze, oblivious to your surroundings, with your eyes fixed only on a far-distant prize.
- Give yourself a break. Your 10k race pace may have slowed to 10 min/mile (it was 8 min/mile as a resident) but at least you are out there running!
- Remember, you are not in your residency or practice simply to get to a certain professional level, to be enjoyed a decade down the line. You are there to live your life in a unique

and amazing setting—one of learning, and personal growth, and drama, and human need, and desperation, and exasperation, and tremendous successes, and tragedies, and gratitude, and hostility. In many ways, you are experiencing an amazingly concentrated version of life, a version that few have the privilege to experience. Soak it in. Reflect upon it. Share it.

> One of our colleagues speaks of putting one's current life in the context of the inevitable future "White Owl" moment. He employs the aphorism "smoking on a White Owl (cigar)" as a euphemism for being on a ventilator in an ICU at the end of life. He proposes, "You know, when I am on my way out, and I am lying there in an ICU, smoking on the ol' White Owl, I don't want to look back on my life with regrets about all that I missed out on. I want to look back with great contentment and realize that I soaked in every last drop of experience and happiness and wonder out of life."

- Remind yourself with some frequency that you have the distinct privilege to lead a life of real meaning. You head to work every day to try to help fellow travelers whose rivers are flowing far faster than yours, whose accelerating waters are full of stumps and rocks and alligators! Your patients are desperately clinging to any lifeline that can slow the process down and offer them a modicum of safety. You are a hero—one who makes the world a safer place for your patients. Embrace it, celebrate it, savor it, and your own current will slow.

CHAPTER TWENTY

I Have Some Good News and…

Hyper-Intense Communications and Delivering Bad News

"The single biggest problem in communication is the illusion that it has taken place."

—*George Bernard Shaw*

"The difference between the right word and the almost–right word is the difference between lightning and the lightning bug."

—*Mark Twain*

The "average" patient today seems sicker than ever before.

> In a survey of our spine clinic (presumably consisting of relatively healthy outpatients), the average patient suffered from 6-10 significant co-morbidities (some more than 15) and was routinely taking 8-12 medications (some up to 20). Ninety percent were overweight, and 50 percent smoked heavily.

When such patients get sick, they get *really* sick. They become very brittle and subject to abrupt and profound deteriorations. They are vulnerable to inexorable downward spirals that can be remarkably difficult to reverse. And, you will find yourself often trying to convey the complexity of it all to people who are distraught and medically unsophisticated. A tall order indeed.

If you are like many physicians, you are often the bearer of bad tidings. In the course of any workweek, you will likely have to discuss with one or many people a new diagnosis of cancer, or a need for a dangerous procedure, or the impending death of a loved one, or the results of a horrible accident, or the serious illness of a child, or a sudden complication in care, or even a mistake in diagnosis or therapy.

What is more, you will be a conduit of important patient and therapeutic information to and for many other members of the healthcare team. You may need to synthesize complex considerations of your specialty for multiple other providers. You may need to convey the urgency of an intervention. You may have to address a mistake or oversight in care. You may need to solicit immediate assistance from other professionals. And, they may not always respond with the urgency, thoughtfulness, and/or intensity that you desire or expect.

You can easily be at the sharp end of the intense communications spear, out there on the healthcare front lines, engaging in multiple crucial conversations with patients, family members, nurses, techs, and other physicians throughout your workdays.

> *We tallied one form of critical conversation engaged in by our residents—discussions with patients or family members about new life-threatening conditions. Our residents averaged over 80 per week, with a maximum of 120!*

Not every intense conversation addresses life-and-death circumstances. People are people, and the simplest of matters can be blown out of proportion or hopelessly misinterpreted. Dangerously, matters that seem trivial to you may be of significant importance to someone else. In such situations, you may fall into the trap of conveying your lack of concern for the matter and set off a powder keg of emotions.

Often, you will find yourself in a no-win conversation. We experience this in our outpatient clinic with great frequency, when patients demand narcotic analgesics or prolonged excuses from work when we don't feel that their conditions warrant them.

> *One of our colleagues, a pediatric orthopedic surgeon, lamented, "I became a surgeon because I love doing surgery—the more complicated and challenging, the better. We are bombarded with complaints from parents of clinic patients who have nothing wrong with them (that surgery can fix). Those parents need a physician who can counsel them and placate them. That's not me!"*

Each critical conversation takes a fair amount of psychic energy. In fact, all medical conversations take a fair amount of psychic energy. They take steeling yourself for a range of reactions. Some will be heartrending and will touch you deeply. Some will be challenging and even abusive. Some will provoke frustration and anger. Others will leave you feeling impotent and without closure. Often, you will have to modify what you are thinking to a more palatable and polite stream of conversation. Each of these exchanges saps your energy reserves. Several such conversations in a row can leave you feeling exhausted and wrung out.

> *One of our colleagues recalls a weekend on call where he had delivered bad news so many times to so many people that he reached his breaking point. With tears in his eyes, he turned to a nearby physician assistant and said, "If I have to tell one more family that their loved one is dead or maimed, I don't think I will make it." Unfortunately, he ended up having to hold several more of these conversations that night. He recalled that he "crawled out of the hospital" Monday morning, canceled a day of clinic, and sat in his backyard and stared at the trees for the entire day.*

Here are a few questions for you to contemplate and discuss with your peers, friends, families, mentors, or perhaps a therapist. Please see www.studergroup.com/thriving-physician for more questions.

Consider and Discuss

- How do you prepare for a difficult conversation with a patient or family?
- Who amongst your team is particularly adept at these types of interactions? What is their secret? Who is not so good? Where do they run into trouble?

- Think about a time when you were on the receiving end of a crucial conversation. How was it handled? How did you feel? How would you have improved it?

- What best restores you after a very intense conversation?

- What are your methods of delivering bad news? Do you wing it? How much preparation for the discussion do you make?

Building Resilience

Realize that critical conversations will take something out of you. If at all possible, give yourself at least a short respite after each one. Don't immediately take on another such conversation or plow into emails or medical records—take a break by going for a short walk outside, or sitting in a quiet area, or listening to some gentle music.

- Don't replay the conversation looking for your mistakes and "I should haves." Rather, focus on something more positive, pastoral, and calming.

- If a conversation was particularly taxing, find a place to sit, sip on some fluids, rest your eyes, and take your mind to a more relaxing place. If none of this is possible, try to drop the aura of the previous interaction prior to entering the next.

- Don't "wing" your crucial conversations. Thoughtfully prepare for them and manage them. Consider upfront what you need to convey, and what you want and need from the conversation. Outline on paper the three most important points you need to get across.

- Anticipate how the person with whom you will have a crucial conversation is likely to respond and what they will want or need from the conversation.

- Practice a crucial conversation in your mind or even role play it with a colleague if you can.

- Always be prepared for a crucial conversation to deviate from how you imagined it might go.

- In a critical conversation, avoid telling yourself a "story" about the motivations behind the other person's responses. Distressed people may act out in many ways, but their intentions are seldom as nefarious as that little voice in the back of your mind may be telling you. Seek to better understand their needs and wants and consider how you might align these with your own.

- Listen. Listen intently. Seek understanding.

- Don't make assumptions. Consider these key words: "What is your understanding of your condition and our plan of care?"
- Recognize that a perfect resolution may not be attainable.

> *Our aforementioned pediatric orthopedic surgeon found relief from the following insight: "I realized recently that I tend to gauge my professional worth with the singular yardstick that 'measures' whether I have done exceptional surgery on a given day or week. I'm learning that if I alter my mindset to match the needs of the patient or patient's parents, I have a different experience. It helps to think,* I do not need to operate here; the definition of good work with this one will be that I have a caring, informative conversation with the parents.*"*

- Try whenever possible to diffuse and de-escalate tension.
- Leverage empathy, a universal connector. The words, "I can imagine how tough this has been for you…" may go a long way to shape a family's perception that you care deeply for their loved one and you are there to help.
- Repeat your message without annoyance. Reflect the conceptualizations of those you are speaking with.
- Don't say anything to the effect of "You are really being unreasonable about this." But also, don't accept abuse.
- Politely end an interaction if it is out of control or abusive. Suggest that you might continue it once you both have a chance to calm down.

Delivering Bad News

Some physicians are highly skilled at delivering bad news and engage in these interactions willfully. Many others "run for the hills." They feel ill-equipped to handle such intense interactions and defer to someone, heck, anyone, else. But the patient's pain is no softer if someone else has to give the news. And, if such news is not going to come from you, the patient's trusted doctor, who will it come from? No one understands the situation better than you.

The good news is that, like so many things, you get better at it with some thoughtfulness and a lot of practice. There is no single right way to break bad news, so we will offer some advice from one of our senior colleagues. He states that he has become an expert in delivering bad news—through no great innate aptitude—but through 35 years of experience in the "warzone" that is tertiary medicine.

He calls his approach **"T.H.E. Cs"**
   T= TOUCH
   H= HONESTY
   E= EMPATHY
   Cs= CONNECTION, COMMAND, COMPETENCE, CONFIDENCE, CLARITY, COMMITMENT, CONSISTENCY, COMPASSION and CARING

Touch—Gently touch the patient at least a couple of times on the shoulder or the forearm or the hand. Touch is so very human and primal. It creates a connection and a bond that words alone cannot reproduce. Warmly shake hands at the beginning and end of the conversation. Hug the patient briefly if they ask or initiate.

Honesty—Sugar-coating won't help a thing and can lead to wildly false hopes and miscommunication of crucial facts, and to the dreaded downstream conversation of "But you said…" So, it is critical to be absolutely forthright and transparent about the situation. This may take some very painful education and explanation, but it must be done. We have found repeatedly that patients and families respond well to total honesty; it creates a bond of trust that will serve the relationship going forward. So be brave, explain the situation clearly, but also as gently and as sensitively as possible.

Empathy—It is okay to feel sad and to grieve with patients and their families to some degree. They will appreciate that you are not cold and detached but that you recognize them as fellow human beings in need. Allow yourself to experience some of their pain and distress. But don't wallow in it—they need you to be clear-eyed and clear-thinking.

Connection—All the concepts in this section help establish a solid doctor-patient connection, at a time when the patient and their loved ones need it the most. Connection is critical in establishing trust, conveying important information, and soothing the patient. If your patients and families feel connected, you can say or do almost anything and not go wrong (even if the words don't come out the way you wanted them to). But your words and concern and gestures must be genuine. Ailing people can sense insincerity in a heartbeat.

Command—All hell is breaking loose for the patient and his or her family. These people depend on you to blaze a trail through a foreign and hostile land. You will need to lead them through these initial very critical conversations, as well as through a potentially protracted, painful, and wrenching series of experiences. This is not the time to be a shrinking violet. So, take command of the situation.

We are not advocating being a dictator here. But you cannot let chaos reign, either. Establish a calm and collected atmosphere for the delivery of the news. Identify those who will best understand the information, those who will support the parties involved, those who are keeping a clear head, and those who the family clearly trust and look up to. If necessary, calmly establish some ground rules of interaction. Sit everyone down and try to find some privacy. Ask the patient and loved ones what they know and understand already. This sets a foundation for the remainder of the discussion and gives you an idea of their medical sophistication.

Competence—The patient and his or her loved ones absolutely must feel you know what you are doing. Otherwise, they will discount most of what you say and may become frustrated, angry, and even hostile. Reassure them that you have been here before. You might establish your credentials and qualifications here: e.g., "I have worked in a stroke unit for the past 15 years," or, "I have performed hundreds of these procedures in my career." Discuss the situation in plain English and in an organized manner exhibiting command of the subject matter, but don't retreat into "medicalese" (the usage of high-level medical terminology).

Confidence—Make it clear that you know what you are talking about, that you are confident in your mastery of the subject and in what you are conveying. This allows the patient and their family to accept that they are receiving the "straight scoop." They need to come out of the discussion thinking that you have given them an absolutely clear picture of what is going on. Be careful of overconfidence, however. You are already in a lofty position in their eyes, so be extremely humble and human. It is very easy for some people to interpret too much confidence and "medicalese" as conceit.

Clarity—This is a big one! All the talking in the world means nothing if your patients don't understand you. We have seen practitioners speak for hours with patients and still not get the message across. Remember, medicine and your specialty have their own languages—languages that the general public does not speak. Slow down, interpret, explain, and teach. Adjust to the level of their medical sophistication. We have found that illustrative similes work well. For example, when speaking about the growth pattern of a brain tumor, we may offer that it is "like a weed with an extensive root system."

Also remember that distressed people do not process information very well. It is likely that little that you convey in a "bad news" conversation will actually get through and hit its mark. Make things straight-forward and orderly. Try to be succinct and to-the-point. Repeat important concepts. Come back and talk further to reinforce the most salient points. Ask directly, "Do you understand?" Solicit clarifying questions. Be straight. Don't beat around the bush to save them some pain or you some discomfort. If you aren't positive that they get it, consider the "teach back" method to validate they can repeat back key information: "Mrs. Jones, would you mind sharing with me what we discussed about the follow-up and next steps in your care?"

Commitment—Be committed to what you are saying; don't waffle or be wishy-washy. If you aren't committed to what you are saying, you will not come off as competent or confident, and you won't be clear. In fact, your audience will stop listening to you.

If the outcome is uncertain, say so directly. But don't vacillate and cloud the issues at hand with your lack of uncertainty. It is okay to be certain about the uncertainty of the situation. Such is the nature of much of medicine. And distressed families are open to acknowledging the mysteries of life. You will connect on a human-to-human level with the patient and family when you say things like the following: "I wish I knew an answer to that," or, "There is only so much all our sophisticated testing can tell us." Furthermore, make sure you show your commitment to your patient. More on this in a bit.

Consistency—Providers often backpedal after "dropping a bomb" of bad news. For example, in order to save a patient/family pain, they may say, "Maybe there is a small chance of an excellent recovery," when they have just said there was not. This helps no one. It creates confusion and makes you come across as being inconsistent in your information delivery and guidance. The second you are perceived as being inconsistent, the family loses faith in your message (often out of wishful thinking). So, express what you truly believe is going on and stick to your guns (it is okay to be wrong at times).

Compassion—Slow down and allow yourself to feel what the patients and their families are going through. Step into their shoes if only for a few moments. Then, "do unto others as you would have done unto you." Treat them with great compassion and understanding. Too many providers try to express compassion without actually feeling it. This is absolutely transparent to the patient/family—even in a time of crisis. It comes off as blindingly false and obsequious. So, if you don't have this skill, learn it!

Caring—Compassion is not conveyed solely through words or hand holding, but rather by demonstrating caring and commitment. Show you are going beyond just empathizing. Demonstrate that you truly care about your patient's plight and are committed to helping them through it. Offer support by asking: *What can I do to help? Is there someone I can call? May I sit with you for a while? Do you want to talk about it more—about how you feel right now? Here is my cell phone number; call me any time.*

Let the patient and their family know that they are affecting you beyond the patient-provider relationship; that you are touched by the humanity of the situation; that they have an ally through their struggles; that you are committed to them. Remember, simple gestures go a long way.

When giving bad news, be prepared for some surprises. No two people react the same way. There will be some anger and possibly even some anger directed at you! But the responses we have experienced the most have been ones of remarkable, almost supernatural, grace. We can cite many examples of extraordinary grace demonstrated by patients and families in the utter worst of times, demonstrated by people of the simplest of means, demonstrated by people of extremely limited emotional reserve. It is a most humbling and almost spiritual experience. Open yourself up to witness such grace, appreciate the humanity of it, soak it in. It will ignite caring and compassion in you. It will inspire you to keep going through some pretty challenging times.

Be careful, though. Breaking bad news takes its toll. We all have a psychological limit to exposure to tragedy and the suffering of others, no matter the grace that is exhibited. Watch yourself. Be aware of when you are feeling depleted.

A Word About Asking for Decisions

Often when delivering bad news, you will be concomitantly in the position of having to ask a patient or family for a decision on therapeutic intervention. These decisions can be massive and urgent, with true life-and-death implications. For example: You are telling a family that their loved one has sustained a massive heart attack and you want to know how aggressive you should be in the patient's management. Be patient and give those involved more time if needed. A few extra minutes to process can alleviate a life of second guessing, remorse, and guilt for decisions made.

Assure those involved that there are no wrong decisions! Make it clear that one answer will not lead to happiness and peace, another to disaster and ruin. So often, these are not "binary" situations. The odds of great outcomes may be extremely limited, the odds of bad things, limitless. Note that it is the situation that is miserable and is in many ways unaffected by whatever decision is made ("the horse is already out of the barn"). Do your best to eradicate downstream guilt and blame for the family members and loved ones. We have seen these scenarios rip families to pieces.

It is okay to offer guidance and gentle direction. You are far more well informed, emotionally insulated, and objective under the circumstances. The concept of "shared decision-making" doesn't necessarily work so well in dire situations, particularly when they are very time-sensitive. Gentle guidance/advice combined with great flexibility may greatly help to alleviate the paralyzing ambivalence that such situations can generate. And remember, emphasize that there are *no wrong decisions*.

CHAPTER TWENTY-ONE

Like Entering a Den of Vipers

Malpractice Litigation

"I think we are faced in medicine with the reality that we have to be willing to talk about our failures and think hard about them, even despite the malpractice system."

—*Atul Gawande*

"America, with 4 percent of the world's population, has 50 percent of the world's lawyers…"

—*Richard Lamm*

All physicians face the specter of hungry plaintiff lawyers, waiting to pounce around the next corner while salivating over every poor patient outcome. Litigation is a fact of life in modern American medicine. It is a major industry backed by very powerful governmental lobbies. Some specialties are affected more than others, but none are immune.

> *Neurosurgeons are sued for alleged malpractice, on average, once every two years. Other specialties that carry the highest likelihood of being sued include thoracic-cardiovascular surgery, general surgery, orthopedic surgery, plastic surgery, obstetrics and gynecology, urology.[1]*

Residents are frequently named in lawsuits although they are seldom brought as far as trial (due to empty pockets). Although malpractice lawsuits are generally not a primary concern for residents, they all know the day is coming when they will be. Residents therefore are certainly not immune to anxiety over litigation vulnerability. We have observed that one of the most common topics of general conversation between residents and their attendings is malpractice litigation.

We regularly run mock malpractice deposition and trial testimony sessions with our residents. Residents play the role of the defendants in cases of bad patient outcome. We employ actual case histories involving patients in whose care the residents intimately participated. The residents face realistic questioning about every facet of the cases. Their notes are dissected. Their decision-making, interventions, commitment, and associated knowledge bases are intensely challenged.

After such role-playing, all residents report that they feel remarkably uncomfortable during these sessions. Yet they feel the sessions are invaluable. They report that even though they recognize that these are exercises, they feel extremely vulnerable and anxiety-ridden, and that these feelings intensify throughout the questioning. They feel they are prevented from representing the truth. They report a sense of being violated, and burn with anger at the injustice of the process.

We have deeply explored with the residents the reasons behind their responses. We point out that they face challenging situations daily, even life-and-death situations, and query what it is about the lawsuit experience that makes them feel so deeply disturbed. They note many reasons. They feel defenseless. They feel that their identities as doctors are under assault. They feel that they cannot possibly win (the care of a complex patient can always be made to look bad). They feel that their expertise is being severely denigrated. They feel guilt for their imperfections and the fact that they actually could have done a better job caring for their patients. They feel like they have no control over the situation. They feel bad for the patients—that the process prevents them from compartmentalizing away thoughts about what happened to their patients.

Hats off to our team for at least touching on the misery that is a malpractice suit. Notification of your suit usually occurs years after the episode(s) of patient care; long after your memory of the associated events has faded. Often it is over a case you never suspected would result in a lawsuit. You may have believed that you had an excellent relationship with the patient and/or their family. You may have thought that things actually went well for the patient. Most times you can't remember much at all of the associated details. And, sadly, your notes will prove to be woefully lacking in the details you now really need to help you mount a formidable defense.

You are treated no differently from those physicians who actually are negligent or malfeasant, who indeed need to be filtered out by the system (and seldom are). You are served with a series of complaints that make you feel like a war criminal. Your records are dissected and your participation denigrated as if you had only one person in the universe to care for, and you royally screwed it up. Your incompetence, negligence, lack of caring, lack of professionalism, lack of expertise are openly asserted, not just implied. You read depositions from professional colleagues declaring under oath (often lying) that everything you did was wrong. You suffer the pain of realizing that some of your actions weren't perfect.

Furthermore, every time you put it out of your mind and refocus on work, family, or fun, the suit resurfaces with more questions from your lawyers and more accusations from the opposition. The process goes on for years. Then the deposition. You are skinned alive by the plaintiff's attorneys. The best you can hope for is to come out of it without making major blunders or "losing it."

Then, if it keeps going, you get to experience the trial. There you learn very quickly that a malpractice trial is not a sophisticated and time-tested system of uncovering the truth and of dispensing appropriate justice. It's essentially just a big show, put on by opposing sides, to win over a jury of medically unsophisticated "peers." There need not be any justice; there need not be any truth. Your odds of "survival" may be no better than those who actually did commit egregious acts of malpractice.

Lies and insults and slander are thrown about you with wanton abandon—often by colleagues from your own specialty. And you have no real recourse. You are trapped in a satellite industry of modern medicine, with very powerful backers. Big money churns away in this industry, and you are a piece of powerless flotsam and jetsam tossed about on its torrid waves.

No wonder research demonstrates that 96 percent of physicians undergoing a malpractice suit acknowledge suffering significant physical and/or emotional struggles during the experience. These include: depression (33 percent), anger (26 percent—this must be an underestimate), physical illness (16 percent), various other painful emotions (13 percent—again, an underestimate), alcohol/drug problems (8 percent).[2]

For many, the pain does not stop at the end of the suit. Many find it hard to return to practice as usual. They narrow the scope of their practices and avoid completely the types of cases that ended in the suit. Not a negligible number leave clinical practice altogether. It is clear that a sizable percentage of physicians suffer from post-traumatic-stress-like syndromes after experiencing a malpractice lawsuit.

Why is the experience so devastating for so many physicians? There are likely a multitude of reasons, many of which were enumerated by our residents.

1. *Control* has to be a major issue. Physicians come to feel that litigation is a spin of the roulette wheel; when our number comes up, we will get sued. We have no control over the who, what, why, where, and when. Win, lose, we have no real role in the outcome.

2. *Fear* of financial and reputational injury is surely a component. Not only could the suit bankrupt us in the present, news of the suit could kill our referral streams and damage our overall careers.

3. *Guilt* rears its ugly head. In review of the records we often have plenty to feel guilty about. Missed diagnoses, imperfect interventions, limited follow-up, missed opportunities to make amends, patient suffering, and abysmal documentation, all pile on.

4. *Sorrow* is a genuine component. Sorrow and worry for the suffering patient and sorrow for oneself having to go through it all.

5. A sense of *violation* runs just beneath the surface. The injustice and lying is so overt and so palpable that we tend to experience the process as a random, wanton, and gratuitous act of emotional violence.

6. *Threat to identity* must also be considered. So much of our persona is defined by our societal role as physicians. Now our competence, dedication, expertise, and intelligence are all called into question. We even have "experts" from our own professional societies weighing in against us.

7. *Grief* is ubiquitous and we must get through multiple phases of it to get to the other side. And not everyone makes it.

But it goes deeper than this. It goes to the physician's very being. Most of us believe that we are truly good, caring, invested, dedicated, loving people. Beyond what society makes of us, we now have to contend with what we think about ourselves: *Maybe I am not the doctor or the person I thought I was.*

Here are a few questions for you to contemplate and discuss with your peers, friends, families, mentors, or perhaps a therapist. Please see www.studergroup.com/thriving-physician for more questions.

Consider and Discuss

- How well are you able to compartmentalize bad or difficult events in your life? Could you do this with all the hullabaloo surrounding a lawsuit?

- What are the rights of a patient who has been injured by medical care or who has an unexpected poor outcome? Does it matter if there was medical error involved? Is someone always at fault? Should someone be accountable? What is fair compensation for the patient? Who should decide?

- What are some constructive responses to a malpractice lawsuit? What can you learn or gain from a lawsuit experience? Could it make you a better doctor?

- How should a physician who practices true negligence be handled? How about an incompetent physician? Is there a "code of silence" among physicians about incompetent colleagues?

- How does a lawsuit affect a physician's relationship with his or her family, friends, medical community, professional organizations, and community? How might these entities affect and be affected by a physician's ways of coping with the lawsuit?

Building Resilience

Ideally, we would all approach a malpractice suit with the attitude "that which doesn't kill me only makes me stronger." After all, there are bad doctors out there who repeatedly hurt patients and should not be in practice. The system is far from perfect, but we have done a very poor job of policing ourselves. So there is not a huge public groundswell behind the elimination of malpractice lawsuits—they simply aren't going away any time soon. But please recognize, we face worse things. The fact of the matter is that a suit won't kill us. Our community won't abandon us. Most of us will not be bankrupted. Most of our patients will neither hear of the suit nor care.

If you do have to face a team of plaintiff lawyers across some shiny mahogany table someday, accept it for what it is. Recognize it is a nightmare world where you cannot win the day and convince them of your supreme competence. They don't care. All you can do is limit damage, and that needs to be your focus.

- Seek to limit the damage to your side of the case. That means limit your answers and don't give anything away. Listen intently to your lawyers. Follow their guidance. You are in foreign and treacherous waters. Your lawyers will know best how to navigate them.

- Protect your persona. Try to separate your "personhood" and professional self-esteem from the suit. This suit is not about who you are—it's about something that happened. These people are in no position to judge your performance. If you believe you did your best—even if you made some mistakes, even if you made some major mistakes—give your ego a complete "bye." A lawsuit is a vile detour from your world of trying to help people in need and should not be allowed to affect your self-belief and your dedication to the profession.

- Remember, a lawsuit is not the forum for exploring how you could have/should have managed the patient better. That is what morbidity and mortality conferences and other peer-review activities are for.

- Don't hesitate to seek peer support and/or counseling. The goal should be to secure a "safe space" where you can freely discuss your thoughts and feelings. This space will likely lie with colleagues who have "been there" themselves. They will be able to offer support, encouragement, reassurance, and coping advice. They can help you develop a "roadmap" of what to expect along the way and how to manage the ups and downs of the process. **Please note:** You must be careful about discussing specific details of a case with colleagues—such discussions are generally "discoverable." Stick predominately to your reaction to it all.

- Remember that a suit is a family affair. Your family will be affected by the stress and the intractability of the process as well.

- Try to continue normal work and family processes despite the stress of this suit. Families of physicians will likely experience periods of resentment toward your colleagues, your community, your profession, and your patients. You too will feel similar resentment. Handle these emotions together as a family. Remember, your family can be a fantastic source of soothing and reassurance—just remember to offer the same back to them.

- With your family and colleagues, develop and espouse philosophies that promote healing, forgiving, and adjusting. Here are a few examples:
  - "This is a difficult but noble profession. We have to face hard things from time to time."
  - "Doctors do make mistakes—this job can never be done perfectly."
  - "It's difficult to be told you've done something wrong when you've tried so hard to do things the right way."
  - "This, too, shall pass."
  - "The goodness that we do in our medical careers far outweighs the pain of this process."
  - "Far and away, most of the patients we have treated have been appreciative and grateful for the care we have given them. We make a positive difference in the world."
  - "I'm not going to be jaded and lose sight of my calling and impact."

- Stay connected! Don't distance yourself from your loved ones out of embarrassment or a misguided sense of protecting them with your silence. Also, they are not the source of your troubles, so resist any temptation to take out your frustrations or anger on them. Fueling anger and resentment within your family will heal no one. Different family members themselves may need different kinds of support at different times. Remember that what's most important when your family goes through a difficult time is how you all come through it. The experience can actually help you all grow closer and deepen mutual respect and gratitude.
- Recognize that everyone handles the experience in their own way and at their own pace. Accept advice and guidance but find the process that feels best to you.
- Don't make the suit your life's work. Stay engaged with your patients, colleagues, and loved ones.
- "Normalize" your responses to the situation by accepting that feelings such as shame, grief, outrage, distress, confusion, victimization, impotence, nihilism, and lack of control are all common and natural responses. Reassure yourself that most of these feelings will calm with time, but will also flare up now and then when the suit invariably reinvades your life.
- Know that malpractice litigation is an occupational hazard, not a condemnation of your professional competence or persona.

- Consider the possibility (no matter how outlandish it may seem) that this experience will actually help you grow and develop further as a physician. It will actually add to your overall professionalism and skills. It may encourage you to truly focus on the needs of your patients, or to be mindful of how you communicate with them, or it may remind you to be more fastidious with documentation.

- Try some *"problem-focused" coping*, in which you invest energies in addressing the actual problem at hand. This might include selecting a good defense lawyer, researching the supporting and contradicting medical literature relevant to the case, helping find defense witnesses, helping your lawyers understand the medicine behind the case, reviewing and critiquing the plaintiff's expert witness testimonies, etc. This may help you satisfy a driving need to participate in a "fixing" activity for the problem.

- Do be careful, though; you can be swallowed up in the process. And, no matter your effort, you can affect only a fraction of the outcome. Recognize that the pace and control over the process can't be mastered by the sheer force of your will or worrying. Seek to control only what you can control.

- Try *emotion-focused coping*, which involves distracting oneself from worry and engaging in healthy self-soothing, support-seeking, and healthy venting. It's counterproductive if not outright harmful to focus endlessly on why a suit happened, what might happen next, or what can be done to solve the problem. These are important considerations, but examining them will take time and clarity of thought. You are more likely to be able to think clearly as the process unfolds if you make time to regularly distract yourself, engage in healthy self-nurturing, and secure support from friends, family, and colleagues.

- Do anything that gives you a reprieve from ruminations about the case. Live a normal life. Play. Enjoy your loved ones.

- Exercise. Regular exercise during a stressful time serves the dual purpose of calming your stress reactions and increasing your sense of control over your world.

- Create a weekly or monthly leisure schedule.

- Practice mindfulness. Each day, try to take conscious note of the aspects of your work and your career that you still enjoy and find meaningful and rewarding.

- Beware of the associated risks of sustaining malpractice litigation. You may find yourself becoming overly cautious in medical practice patterns (e.g., refusing to treat difficult cases, or specific types of patients), considering early retirement, giving up medicine altogether, being obsequious with your patients, disrupting doctor-patient rapport by spending excessive time obsessing on details or on "cover your tracks" documentation, becoming overly sensitive to perceived slights or criticism, withdrawing from colleagues or family, self-medicating with alcohol or other drugs, or questioning your own spirituality or faith. All are normal responses but are maladaptive. They can easily lead to great dissatisfaction, disaffection, and trouble.

- Be very aware of digging yourself into a deeper legal hole. If a mistake was made, or sub-optimal care was indeed at the heart of the suit, don't try to bury the truth. This will lead only to greater problems downstream. Firstly, overt lying could create a criminal case (perjury) out of a civil one. More importantly, it creates a situation where your self-identity comes under "auto-assault." You have others shooting away at your integrity; now you have given yourself ample opportunity and reason to fire upon it yourself. On a more practical note, if a manipulation of the truth is discovered, it will kill your defense, even if your defense had significant merit.

- If the suit unmasks a real deficiency in your skill set, there are ways to mitigate the situation going forward: courses, seminars, mini-apprenticeships. It is healthy to use the advent of a suit to reexamine your professional competencies. Just beware of judging yourself too harshly under the duress of the process. Turn to trusted colleagues and ask for honest assessment.

- Realize that, in your day-to-day practice, you have more control over risk than you realize (although it will never be total). Appropriate documentation and proper patient engagement and communication have been demonstrated to significantly reduce the risk of suit, even in the face of profoundly poor outcomes. Most hospital risk management departments have abundant materials and seminars on risk amelioration, as do many specialty professional societies. Invite your risk management professionals to meet with you and your team on a regular basis.

- Get involved in risk and quality committees in your institution.

- Attend various root cause analysis meetings to learn to recognize potential flashpoints in patient care.

- Consider having your system's malpractice defense lawyers come speak with your team.

- Role play with colleagues difficult patient interactions and even mock depositions.

- Ask colleagues to share with your group their own litigation experiences. Respectfully analyze these experiences for what can be learned both about risk avoidance and coping with the lawsuit process.

CHAPTER TWENTY-TWO

When We Are the Problem

Abusive Physician Behavior (and the Abused Child Syndrome)

"There are generally three parties to child abuse: the abused, the abuser, and the bystander."
—Louise Penny

"A human being born into a cold, indifferent world will regard his situation as the only possible one."
—Alice Miller

We firmly believe that the majority of physicians are superlative individuals who give deeply of themselves. As humans, however, each of us runs the risk of burning out and imbuing our trainees, subordinates, and even colleagues with some bad conceptualizations, habits, and behaviors. We will all make mistakes. We will at times act out, or make comments that we wish we had not, or snap, or make inappropriate jokes. But every maladaptive action affects others negatively. Some acts hurt people directly. Others set an example of unwanted behavior that the impressionable actually go on to emulate.

For most of us, these are lapses that happen when our defenses are down, when we are emptied out. We recover and return to being reasonable, interactive, community-oriented beings. Amongst us, though, are some truly damaged individuals who are capable of inflicting true, sustained harm upon those they touch.

Physicians are the progeny of a long line of professional predecessors, many of whom justifiably earned the reputation of being uniquely unpleasant. Whether an auto-selection process came into play, or the world of medicine molded (warped?) them, successive generations have been rife with some singularly disagreeable characters. All the old timers will recall, almost with a twisted relish, the tyrants with whom they had to contend during their careers.

> *Stories abound of how residents at one renowned program took call every other night (with no ensuing day off). The chairman of the program was known to stalk the hospital hallways in the middle of the night. If he discovered an on-call resident sleeping, the resident was fired on the spot.*

Family systems research supports the notion that those raised in abuse are more prone to go on and abuse than those who were not.[1] The same seems to be true for battered physicians. Scattered throughout the hospital systems of modern medicine still reside the ogres, the screamers, the abusers, the belittlers, the demeanors, the soul-suckers, the cruel, the remonstrative, and those who derive ego succor from the deconstruction of others.

> *One of our colleagues recalls how rounds began at 5:30 every morning at his training program. One very snowy morning, he showed up 15 minutes late after digging out his pregnant wife's car from a drifted snow bank. Upon hearing about the resident's tardiness, an attending surgeon spent half an hour screaming at the resident in front of the entire service and threatening to fire him if such an occurrence were to happen again.*

Stories still abound of all sorts of abuse. It need not be as overt as excessive and loud rebukes or threats of termination. We hear not infrequently of faculty physicians who pressure and expect their trainees to lie about hours worked (violating the ACGME 80-hour rule), to cover for an attending's inaccessibility on call, to share authorship of original written work to which the attending had not contributed, or to fudge on research results. We are all also cognizant of physicians who blame subordinates for their own complications, even when the subordinates were merely spectators in the therapeutic interventions.

Even more subtle forms of abuse are common and can erode the victim's energies, emotional stability, and resilience. Witness the physician who makes all subordinates stick around the hospital for endless evening rounds, the physician who uses subordinates as personal assistants—"go take my wife to the airport," the surgeon who will not perform a certain type of procedure unless there is a resident to "assist" (i.e., the resident is the only one in the room competent to perform the procedure), the physician who is incapable of ever warmly greeting a subordinate, and so on.

Here are a few questions for you to contemplate and discuss with your peers, friends, families, mentors, or perhaps a therapist. Please see www.studergroup.com/thriving-physician for more questions.

Consider and Discuss

- What behaviors by your superiors or colleagues are you openly or privately vowing to never replicate? Of these vows, which ones have eroded as you have scaled the hierarchical ladder?

- How often do you treat your subordinates poorly? How often have you been outright abusive? What circumstances make it more likely that you will mistreat a subordinate?

- What do subordinates need most from you? How aware are you of how you affect those under you? Do you know what they truly think of you? Do they feel safe and comfortable around you? Would they give you honest feedback if you solicited it?

- How do you feel if you snap at a resident? A colleague? A physician from another specialty? A nurse?

- Have you ever addressed colleagues whom you have witnessed abusing subordinates? What level of abuse would precipitate such a response? Should it be a lower level than that?

Building Resilience

The cycle of arbitrary abuse of junior staff, residents, medical students, and allied healthcare workers will not end unless and until we all take an active role in shaping a positive workplace culture. If you went through a particularly gruesome training experience, try to remember the sheer misery of it all, and vow not to repeat it. This will take a good deal of reflection, self-awareness, self-correction, and more. Consider soliciting feedback from those under you and accept it constructively and without retribution. Seek support and guidance if you find yourself slipping into abusive behaviors.

Be honest and forthright in your discussions with your peers about this issue. Acknowledge that your relationships with each other and with coworkers will be a driving force in either your resilience or your emotional distress and burnout. Be honest about your roles. Virginia Beeson of The Advisory Board Company reminds us that an abusive workplace requires "cooperation" between at least four categories of players:

- The Actors: those whose behaviors are distressing, disruptive, or disrespectful of others.
- The Bystanders: those who remain passive, normalize and/or work-around the disruptive behavior of others, and generally assume an "it's not my job to confront this" stance.
- The Enablers: those whose action or inaction "authorizes" the disruption.
- The Collaborators: those who preserve and perpetuate the disruptive culture.

Remember, all under you are extremely vulnerable and exquisitely sensitive to your attitude and behavior. They crave and need your guidance, kindness, empathy, understanding, and affirmation. This does not mean that tough love cannot be employed when needed. But realize that it will be experienced far more intensely than you intend or perceive.

> One of our colleagues noted that she had seen herself as being jovial, care-free, nurturing, understanding, and perpetually kind with her residents. Through a series of resident surveys and interviews, she found out that the residents perceived her as being inconsistent in mood (often angry), seldom complimentary, and very intimidating. She was dumbfounded. This was not her perception of herself at all. She immediately set out to try to correct these behaviors.

- Make it a point to compliment and give as much positive feedback as possible to those under you.
- Notice the accomplishments of those under you. Be willing to tell them you are proud of their work and their growth.
- Share the glory with those under you when your team acquires various accolades.

- Be on the lookout for abusive behavior in yourself. You may not be recognizing it. Solicit opinions from those around you.

- When disappointed or upset with those under you, hold your tongue for a minute and think of how to constructively guide them to better behavior or performance.

- Seek to make those under you feel safe and respected in your presence. Be their hero, not their tormentor. A hero is someone who makes those around him or her feel safe and valued.

- Be on the lookout for abusive behavior in your colleagues. If you become aware of it, seek constructive, non-threatening, and non-judgmental ways of discussing it with them. "Hey, Frank, young Dr. Smith seemed pretty crestfallen after you last spoke with him. How do you think he took your discussion?"

- Overt and harmful abuse should be addressed directly but may require frank discussion with your chain of command and institutional corrective action.

- Be on the lookout for abusive behavior in those under you. Remember, the slippery slope to being a jerk can start early in training—when the fresh-faced, naïve medical and allied health students come onto your service. Nip such behavior in the bud.

CHAPTER TWENTY-THREE

Trying to Fit a Square Peg into a Round Hole

Finding Your Own Path in the Medical World

"Human tragedies: We all want to be extraordinary and we all just want to fit in. Unfortunately, extraordinary people rarely fit in."

—*Sebastyne Young*

"I may be the wrong person for my life."

—*Thomas McGuane*

When you began your first day of residency training, you had already come through a series of stringent filters purportedly assuring the very best candidate for the job. And supposedly, the job was tailored for your likes, needs, and aptitudes. But is this truly the case? Are you in the right profession? The right specialty? The right subspecialty? The right group? The right healthcare system? The right location?

The filters for entry into medicine are rather unidimensional. Traditionally, they have favored those with the ability, drive, and obsessiveness to memorize huge volumes of data. Cognitive flexibility and critical thought have generally not been emphasized in the selection process.

Think of the ultimate pre-med filter: organic chemistry. Here is a subject that has essentially no relevance to your day-to-day practice of medicine but has traditionally been the master key to unlocking a medical future. At least as taught to undergraduates, organic chemistry is not an intuitive discipline requiring a multi-staged, layered, and flexible thought process. Rather, it is a collection of facts that must be memorized, only to be disgorged later on one or two exams. This process is rather anachronistic nowadays when almost every scientific and medical fact is accessible through the swipe of a screen on a handheld electronic device. Organic chemistry favors those willing to grind out the memorization in order to secure a position at the top end of the bell-shaped curve. You know this; you did it! We all did it!

Of course, it is true that that "organic" is a relatively good predictor of success in medical school. The reason? What is needed to succeed in medical school is quite similar to what is needed to make it through organic chemistry. Medical school, as you remember, involves the memorizing of an infinite collection of often unrelated factoids. There is nothing in either organic chemistry or medical school that is particularly difficult to conceptualize or figure out. But there is memorization, and even more memorization. The more thorough the memorization, the better your medical school grades and board scores, and the more attractive you become to residency programs.

Now comes "the rub." Whilst your memorization of oodles of facts is critical to building an infrastructural foundation in the medical discipline of your choosing, the practice of the discipline itself requires synthesis of the facts and their integration into a multi-dimensional, hyper-variable, ever-changing, and hyper-complex medical real world. Now, critical thinking and hyper-adaptable thinking (street smarts), as well as emotional intelligence and interactive intelligence, are of equal or greater importance.

For example, when trying to decide whether an acutely paralyzed patient has a true neurological disorder or is malingering, memorized facts of nervous system function will help you, but will not determine the final answer. When a child is in your emergency room with a possible acute abdomen, there is rarely a single diagnostic test that will tell you yea or nay about whether to operate. When a medical patient with a dozen significant comorbidities is "crashing" on the ward, hyper-adaptable thinking rather than memorized facts is more likely to get you (and the patient) out of the situation.

But who have we weeded out in the medical school and residency selection processes? Potentially those who would excel at the hyper-variable dynamic of modern medicine—those who are multi-dimensional, well-rounded, interpersonally perceptive, culturally/socially aware, emotionally intelligent, articulate and comfortable in conversation, collaborators, team players, those who are empathically oriented to others, those who value humor and social bonds, and those with true "street smarts."

> One of our medical colleagues recalls two friends from college who were "filtered out" of the medical school chase—both brilliant—both caring, concerned, kind, considerate, intuitive, and "fast on their feet." Both, he insists, would have made wonderful and contributing physicians. Both received "Cs" in organic chemistry and dropped out of pre-med studies. Both went on to take the LSATs and the GMATs. BOTH scored in the 99th percentiles in each exam (so much for their intellectual insufficiency).
>
> One, when asked in a law school application question to "describe your greatest attribute," responded, "brevity." Harvard Law was insightful enough to snatch him up.
>
> The other, when asked in a business school application to "explain the reason for any sub-par grades you might have in your transcripts" responded, "There were occasions when I felt it was more beneficial to my personal growth to have a beer with friends, than to hole up in the library stacks and cram more economics." He was accepted to the Wharton, Chicago, Stanford, and Harvard Business Schools.
>
> Would not the field of medicine have prospered with the mirth of the first and the transparency of the second?

Despite fairly universal agreement on the desirability of diversity in our programs, one risk of our selection and training process is that we are hewing down the pre-med and medical school fields to a fairly uniform type of being (with reference to cognitive processing qualities, at least).

The rough and tumble world of medicine is particularly challenging to many physicians. The ever-changing landscape of the discipline seems to be particularly stressful to those who are used to the orderly processing of data, those who were rewarded their whole academic lives for perfectionistic linear thought, those who are not used to thinking on their feet.

Another important aspect of fit concerns personality type and psychological style. How well can an intensely private and introverted person function in a specialty that requires near constant and intense interaction with patients and families? How well will an extrovert and conversationalist fare in a specialty that locks him or her away in the dark bowels of a hospital studying slides or computer screens? Combine various learning styles with various personality sets, and the matching of trainees to their ideal specialties may go far beyond what is lucrative or conducive to work/life balance or "sexy." Perhaps the specialty selection process could use an in-depth analysis of these components.

And fit does not stop here. We have seen great physicians who thrive in their subspecialties careen off the tracks when paired with the wrong partners, wrong practices, or wrong healthcare systems. We have seen families implode when they situate themselves in regions totally void of family and friends and/or foreign to their geographic and climatic proclivities.

The message is clear: Finding the place you belong in the medical community is crucial not only to your success but to your personal level of career satisfaction and resilience as well.

Here are a few questions for you to contemplate and discuss with your peers, friends, families, mentors, or perhaps a therapist. Please see www.studergroup.com/thriving-physician for more questions.

Consider and Discuss

- What do you think are the key psychological traits or characteristics necessary for success in medical training? Are they the same traits that make for a "good" practicing physician? How would you screen for these traits?

- Does the medical world feel like a constant strain to you or a "smooth ride"? Do you have to change your basic self to fit into the physician "model"? Does caring for others and interacting with others truly make you happy?

- What course in college would be a good predictor for the eventual production of an excellent physician? What extracurricular activities? What type of exam? What interview questions?

- Have you ever taken a personality inventory or psychological style inventory? Do you know what type of personality grouping you fall under? What are the strengths and challenges of your personality type? How does it fit with your specialty and medicine in general?

- Are you in the right specialty? Subspecialty? Practice group? Hospital system? Healthcare system? Part of the country?

Building Resilience

We are not purporting that the great medical educational machinery misfired when it selected you, or any of us. We do question, however, whether "one size fits all" in medicine. If your learning style and personality clash with the demands of your selected specialty, or if your value system and preferred practice style clash with the group you have joined, you may be subject to a life of inordinate stress.

- It is worth spending some time considering how you feel within your specialty and within your practice or organization? Are the intellectual challenges invigorating or exhausting? Do you feel constantly behind the curve or like you are riding the crest of the wave? One warning here. We see over and over again our residents feeling overwhelmed by it all in their first few years. Then, somewhere around PGY 3 or 4, something seems to click for most, and it all seems so much easier. So, give it some time before you assume you've landed in the wrong place in the medical universe.

- Being a great physician is hard, and it takes hard work no matter your fit. But the struggle should still feel energizing or at least stimulating. If it is not, stop, consider, and examine your interface with your chosen field. Do the intellectual demands fit your learning style and capabilities? Can you organize the material you must master such that it fits your learning style? Do the interactive demands fit your personality? Are you truly interested in what you are experiencing and learning?

- If you answered "no" in either category, can you adapt? Are you simply in the wrong training program? Are there sub-specialty tracts within the specialty that will better fit who you are? For example, an ER physician who finds he or she receives no positive "vibes" from the acute care of adults may find that he or she derives a tremendous thrill from pediatric emergency care.

- If you find yourself absolutely miserable within your specialty over a prolonged period of time (everyone is subject to situational depressions and mood swings), it does not mean you are a failure. It most likely means that you ended up in a specialty or a work setting that is a poor fit for your natural psychological and vocational strengths and preferences.

If this is the case for you, please don't feel you are trapped within the discipline. It is okay to consider changing specialties. Or changing jobs. It is even okay to consider getting out of medicine altogether, although the field is so diverse in its needs that almost every learning style and personality can fit nicely into some framework (there are physicians who have found tremendous satisfaction in the realms of administration or quality control or insurance services, for example).

> *We have known many residents and practicing physicians who realized that their chosen specialties did not work for them. They eventually left their original field and went into related disciplines. All reported back to us exceptional job satisfaction in their new disciplines.*

- Likewise, survey the other components to fit. It is so very common for physicians and their families to totally uproot and sever critical friendship, family, and geographic ties, every step along the way of the medical career continuum (e.g., home to undergraduate education to medical school to residency to fellowship to initial job to second job to higher profile job to chairmanship job, etc.). Most moves are based strictly on the medical training and job descriptions with no attention paid to the distance from friends and family, geographic qualities, compatibility with our new colleagues, social opportunities and compatibility for our family members, employment opportunities for our life partners, comfort with the new practice model, or compatibility with the new hospital/healthcare system. These are critical factors that should absolutely enter your education/job calculations. This can be a tall order, however. Generally, you end up grabbing desperately the rung of the next step up on the medical career ladder without fully considering the consequences (or having any other choice). Making career changes based on "fit" may require finding the courage to adjust your career course to better align with your deepest values.

> *We know a physician who took a $500,000 yearly pay cut in order to leave a group filled with interpersonal acrimony and join a group whose norms of professionalism better matched her own. At last report: "I do sometimes miss the money. On the other hand, I count the blessings daily for the more-than-ample income that I do have, and for the happiness and satisfaction that my career has brought to me and my family. Leaving that first group is one of the things I've done in my life that I am proudest of."*

We advise carefully considering all these components if at all possible in your journey along your medical career. If you find yourself desperately chaffing, consider all of these factors: You are not immune to longing for the closeness of your family and friends. You are not immune to desperately missing the familiar surroundings of your home geography. You are not immune to feeling cheapened by a system that pushes you too hard for productivity.

Fit on so many fronts is critical. Find it, and you will cruise. Miss it, and you may never feel comfortable or satisfied.

CHAPTER TWENTY-FOUR

Great Expectations

Unrealistic Patient Expectations and Angry Patients

"Your most unhappy customers are your greatest source of learning."

—*Bill Gates*

"It is not the employer who pays the wages. Employers only handle the money.... It is the customer who pays the wages."

—*Henry Ford*

Despite huge advances in technological and pharmacological support, and refinement of medical and surgical interventions, the delivery of healthcare is often fraught with poor or limited outcomes. In obstetrics, babies still are born with cerebral palsy. In oncology, people still succumb to pancreatic cancer. In cardiology, people still develop debilitating or fatal congestive heart failure. In our field, neurosurgery, even with exquisite and successful procedural interventions, we watch helplessly as many of our aneurysm-rupture patients die, or are maimed by their disease. And so on.

Meanwhile, television and movies depict startling recoveries from the most sensational of diseases, often at the hands of physicians of unrelated specialties!

We doctors don't make it any easier on ourselves either. Caught up in the competitive nature of modern medicine, we are not immune to exaggerating the efficacy of our interventions. We are all to one degree or another culpable in promoting an "expectation inflation." We advertise, sometimes overtly and other times more subtly, our superiority to other providers and other centers. We crow about new technologies and depict routine exceptional results. The net effect is patient anticipation of superlative outcomes—outcomes that may be startlingly divergent from reality.

Beyond this, patients often come armed with a wealth of Internet-derived information about their conditions and sky-high expectations. Only, the "information" is often inaccurate. Purported outcomes are often overgeneralized or out-and-out fallacious. Furthermore, patients may be carrying notions about a related or similar, but not the same, condition as their own.

Now you, the physician, must not only educate patients about their conditions, but also must counter their preformed (and often quite fixed) conceptualizations about their situations. You may spend inordinate time and effort reinforcing the realities of their interventions and explaining the disparity between expected and actual outcomes. Given how desperately many patients and family members cling to hope, even the most extensive pre-interventional counseling may not alter the patients' expectations (and eventual disappointment).

At times you may feel "backed into a corner" in your counseling. You may become concerned that if you do not paint a rosy and hopeful picture, patients are likely to become angry, seek their care elsewhere, rate you poorly on various websites and surveys, become litigious, or all of the above.

What is more, patients indeed seem quick to anger these days. The status, trust, and admiration bestowed upon our medical forefathers by their patients seems a thing of the past. Instead, a begrudgingly shared and suspicious temporary stewardship over a patient's condition is often today's reality. The most minimal inconsistency in care, or tardiness for an appointment, may precipitate a response of invectiveness and vitriol. And any perceived slight (perhaps about weight or smoking habit) may have the same effect.

And when a patient's course goes poorly—no matter the circumstances—watch out! Patients feel as betrayed as if there has been an intentional and overt breach of contract. Many discussions end up in the most uncomfortable and unprofitable pantomime of you feeling compelled to respond to the patient's anger rather than focus on the facts and needs at hand. Even the best of interactions can leave both parties maximally ill at ease and distrustful, with a bucket of unresolved issues.

If you are a resident, you are particularly vulnerable in this "expectation vs. outcome trap." You are perpetually on the "front lines"—rounding frequently on all the most involved patients. You are the first to be called when a patient is upset or requires a clarification or explanation. You are the first on the scene when a complication occurs. You are quickly identified by nurses, patients, and patient families as the spokesperson for the entire team.

Despite all this, you are still a trainee. You lack experience handling these types of conversations, and you lack overall clinical experience—particularly with complications. Thus you often enter into these critical conversations a step behind. You have yet to develop a set point of interaction between the brutally honest and the reassuring. You are often "flying by the seat of your pants"—something that patients or family members may detect and react to.

Here are a few questions for you to contemplate and discuss with your peers, friends, families, mentors, or perhaps a therapist. Please see www.studergroup.com/thriving-physician for more questions.

Consider and Discuss

- Which sorts of patient expectations are most difficult for you to deal with? How do you deal with them? How do you deal with the unrealistic expectations of others (family, friends, coworkers)?

- Do you ever become angry with your patients? How do you handle this? Are there better ways? How do you feel afterwards?

- How can one be brutally honest yet reassuring for a patient?

- How much does a patient absorb in counseling sessions? How can this be improved upon?

- How much is "too much information" when counseling a patient?

Building Resilience

As we alluded to in our opening quotations, there is great value in viewing your patients as customers, and to seeing your practice or your institution as a business, in fact, as a **service industry**. No business can survive if it does not seek to please its customers. No business can thrive without really pleasing its customers. Granted, medicine has unique qualities that separate it from the typical businesses, such as "customers" who are in potentially big trouble, dire associated circumstances, potentially horrific ramifications of poor performance, and a massive surrounding industry that is forever altering and intervening in your efforts. Such differences, however, should only make the desire to please the customer more intense.

All too often, we in medicine become so harried and so multi-tasked that we lose sight of what it is all about: the care of people in distress. We become numb to the situations our customers are in and their responses to them. Why shouldn't a person facing cancer read everything there is on the Internet about their condition, question you about their care, respond suspiciously to inconsistencies and knowledge gaps, and express fear, frustration, and anger?

- The key here is to understand the lot of your patient; to walk a mile in their shoes; to forgive anxiety, stress, anger, and even rudeness; and to reset your own expectations. Patient interactions will never be akin to conversations with buddies about sports or idle chitchat. These will always be "crucial conversations." These will always be supercharged and intense. So much rides on them for your patients.

- Staying resilient requires well-developed emotional intelligence, a combination of self-insight, self-regulation, empathy, interpersonal sensitivity, and capacity for influencing others. Thus, when interacting with patients and their families, you need to be aware of your own response to their situations and reactions. How do you feel when a patient is anxious, frustrated, sad, or angry? Do your own feelings color your response? How can you alter your responses by acknowledging the feelings patients create in you?

- The next step is to consider how you might better please patients (customers) in their various states. It won't be the same for every patient in every situation. This will not always mean a therapeutic "win." Often it may mean something entirely different from a therapeutic outcome. You may need to redefine what a "good enough" outcome of this consultation will be.

You may not be able to give patients what they want (e.g., relief from chronic pain, medication that is not indicated, or a cure). Yet you can ask yourself: *What is something I can realistically do to put this patient more at ease? Even if I cannot alleviate all of their suffering, what can I do to calm their ruminations and bring them a modicum of hope? How might I dissipate some of their anger? How can I educate them? How can I help them face their fears?*

> One of our very successful colleagues, who seems universally loved by his patients, described his method of relating to them: "I had to teach myself to like my patients—all of my patients. This meant never making judgments about them—just like them. When you like someone, you do everything you can to help them and make them happy."

We encourage you to take our colleague's great advice, for your own sake as well as for your patients. Negative emotions (no matter how "justified" they may be) erode personal resilience. Too often we are quick to blame our patients for poor interactions, when the real cause is our failure to make our customers happy. But if we remember that they are likely frightened and intimidated and confused (and frustrated by our oft-imperfect healthcare "systems"), perhaps we can return to liking them and focusing on their needs. We can let our humanity drive the ship. We can provide the best "customer service" possible because it is the right thing to do.

Remember, *meaning is the antidote to burnout*. Pleasing a patient who is in the middle of difficult times is inherently meaningful (or should be). Isn't this really what you went into medicine to do? The better you become at it, the more you will reconnect with the inner motivations of practicing medicine. The work may be harder, but it will be vastly more rewarding. Furthermore, liking and enjoying your patients will shorten the day, make the work less of a drudgery, and make the workday less lonely.

- Remind yourself that the patient sitting there in your exam room is a customer. Seek to understand what they are looking for in this exchange. Don't be afraid to ask them directly (e.g., "What can I do to help you today?").
- Resist telling yourself a story about the motivations of your patients. Take them at face value.

- Be honest when you cannot deliver exactly what they want. Seek to give them close to what they want whenever possible. This is as often emotional support as it is actual medical administrations.

- Put away any judgments about your patients predicated on appearance, educational level, insurance, work history, hygiene, social skills, etc. Focus on what they are looking for from you.

- Always offer the patient a good dose of humanity and treat them with great dignity. Doing this will please the grand majority of your "customers."

- Connect with your patients. Make eye contact, sit down, examine them (even if just superficially), smile, speak clearly (avoid "medicalese") but not down to them, focus on them (and not all your other distractions), thank them for coming to see you.

CHAPTER TWENTY-FIVE

But You Said…

Realistic Patient Expectations

"Achievement is largely the product of steadily raising one's levels of aspiration and expectation."
—*Jack Nicklaus*

"Don't lower your expectations to meet your performance. Raise your level of performance to meet your expectations. Expect the best of yourself, and then do what is necessary to make it a reality."
—*Ralph Marston*

Even though we cannot all stride through our hospitals blithely dispensing miracles, medicine has remarkably (almost miraculously) progressed over the past several decades. It has blossomed with respect to treatment efficacy, applied technology, and patient safety. We have come a long way in medical and surgical outcomes—across all specialties.

Thanks to the widespread dissemination of medical information through the Internet and other media, many patients are quite aware of this progress. Thus, they come to their physicians well informed and expecting state-of-the-art care. This creates an immediate challenge. The honest physician may wonder: *Am I the right doctor for this patient? Can I contribute to this patient's care as well as other doctors? Is my hospital or healthcare system the right one to best care for this patient?*

Consider the dilemma of surgeons facing particularly challenging procedures. The moral surgeon surely deals internally with the fact that, no matter what the procedure, another surgeon somewhere can perform a specific operation better. This may be particularly a concern for "proceduralists," but it really applies to all providers. There is always someone out there who can "do the job better," no matter the medically related activity.

Patients rightfully expect outcomes that at least approximate accepted specialty norms. This means that every physician, including you, is expected to clinically bring his or her "A-game" to the medical "playing field" on a daily basis. You do not have the luxury of doing only a "passable" job. You were used to excelling in everything during your scholastic career. Now you find out that this level of performance is expected of you for the rest of your life. This can be rather exhausting.

But it is not just in clinical performance that you are expected to excel. Patients rightfully expect you to be accessible, and available, and affable, and well informed, and patient, and interested, and communicative, and engaged. This is often at odds with your busy schedule. You may have appointment and procedural-scheduling backlogs of weeks or even months. Outpatient visits may be limited to a few minutes of "quality" interactive time (with the rest soaked up by EMR charting, narcotic use checks, filling out forms, etc.). You may have to count on physician assistants and nurse practitioners to carry out a significant portion of your practice's outpatient visits, thus further limiting your interactions with your patients.

For these reasons, you may deal with nagging guilt and the "impostor syndrome": "I am pretending to be a doctor, but am I really being one?"

If you are a resident, you are caught in a particular bind. You have no control over the situation, yet you are one of the team members with the greatest amount of interaction with the patients. You will field their frustrations and disappointments. You will often have to explain and apologize for the attending physicians' and the system's shortcomings. You will feel you have to protect your team and project an aura of institutional superiority. You will be responsible for much of the patients' interventional counseling. You will be required to discuss intricacies of interventions you may have little experience in. If anyone begins to feel like an imposter, it will be you.

Here are a few questions for you to contemplate and discuss with your peers, friends, families, mentors, or perhaps a therapist. Please see www.studergroup.com/thriving-physician for more questions.

Consider and Discuss

- What exactly is involved in a "contract between a patient and his or her physician"?

- What do you expect out of physicians who care for you? How does this compare with what your patients expect of you and what you give to your patients?

- Is it possible to meet all of your patients' expectations and needs? How close must you get? How do you do so? How do you reconcile the disparity?

- Imagine yourself as a patient on the service. Knowing all that you know, what would be your expectations? What "special care" would you request/demand/expect? What would constitute the perfect interface with your providers and the perfect course of care?

- Are you honest with yourself about your own capabilities? Are you honest with your patients? Can you list what in your field you are best at and what you are worst at?

Building Resilience

Patients have a right to expect you to be truly competent in your field and to know when you are overreaching. But this is the "stuff" of all that you learned in your schooling and training. You excel at this—that is why you are where you are. Recognize that while there will always be people with greater expertise and skill than you, this does not make you an imposter. You can never master it all, but you can be a lifetime learner who constantly strives to improve. You certainly should not be one who rests on your laurels and fails to grow in your career.

- If you are a trainee, resilience will require you to constantly stretch your comfort zone to gain new competencies. But remaining resilient as a practicing physician requires a twist to this strategy: recognizing and working around your limitations. These are the things that you have little aptitude or appetite for. When you have the option, eliminate or delegate those areas from your career palette. This is where a team approach is useful. Finding partners who are strong in areas where you are weak is a career survival skill. It is okay to steer particularly challenging cases their way. Ideally, such behavior will be reciprocated, and you will know you are doing what is best for your patients. If need be, steer a patient to a true national expert outside of your system. And do so without shame or guilt. Remember: None of us can be great at everything.

- Meeting patient expectations for your availability, length of time in consultations, complete undivided attention, and so on, is a bit more of a "sticky wicket." You simply will not have the time or needed personnel to provide such care. This dynamic will persist throughout your career, and there will always be some patients who want more of your time than you can deliver. In these situations, we advocate being open and honest with your patients about your time constraints and availability.

- The most difficult resilience lesson for most physicians is learning to set limits and to have appropriate boundaries when responding to the endless needs of those they serve. Setting such limits does not mean you have to be inflexible or dismissive. Rather, learn to caringly and compassionately underscore your many obligations. Reinforce that you do all you can to be fair to all of your patients. A simple statement like, "I wish I had more time available to visit with you" will go a long way in softening the limit that you are setting.

> *It doesn't always work. One of our family practice colleagues was scolded for missing (postponing) an appointment with one of his fibromyalgia patients. He rescheduled her appointment for the same week. Upon greeting her, he expressed regret at having to cancel her appointment at the last minute and openly apologized. He explained that a young renal patient he had been following in the hospital had deteriorated rapidly and required an emergent intervention. But, the fibromyalgia patient maintained that our colleague had abandoned her, and should have left the inpatient's care to one of his partners. He explained that the inpatient had invested his trust in him and desperately needed him at the time. The lady responded, "Well, so did I." And, in a manner, she was correct. Sometimes, all you can do is what you think is your best!*

- As a trainee, the more you pour yourself into the intricacies and science of your specialty, the broader the scope you will feel competent to cover.

- As a practicing physician, staying a student of your field will likewise bear fruit. National meetings and courses are worth your time on multiple fronts.

- Dedicate a small amount of time each day to read your trade journals. Perusing an article or two a day is far more effective than trying to catch up on six months' worth of your journals.

- Learn something new about anything that makes you anxious. This is a sure way to soothe your anxieties (at least a bit) and increase your efficacy for dealing with that very thing.

- Periodically list your strongest and your weakest clinical competencies. Resilience entails coming to terms with your own strengths and limitations. If you are weak in certain areas—and if you deem it important to do so—put the time and effort into mastering them! Do some extra reading or attend special courses. Grant yourself permission to seek out and learn from teammates who excel in areas that you do not.

- Beware of so-called "avoidance" coping strategies—doing everything other than engaging in the activity that generates anxiety. When facing areas that make you uncomfortable, these behaviors only fuel anxiety, and this anxiety erodes your resilience. Intense focus on whatever is bothering you tends to yield satisfaction and "shrinks" the effect of the stressor.

- Go out of your way to make each patient feel that the time spent with you was real, interactive, and worthwhile.

- If you must enter information into an EMR during the visit, break your attention away from the computer and look directly at the patient intermittently. Allow them to talk uninterrupted about their problems and needs for at least a couple of minutes.

- Make sure you touch your patients, either by some form of examination or by placing a reassuring hand on a shoulder or arm.

- Ask pointed questions that demonstrate you listened to your patients' concerns. Reflect back to them what you understand about their concerns.

CHAPTER TWENTY-SIX

Living in a Digital World

The Supremacy of the Electronic Medical Record

"Electronic medical records are, in a lot of ways, I think the aspect of technology that is going to revolutionize the way we deliver care. And it's not just that we will be able to collect information; it's that everyone involved in the healthcare enterprise will be able to use that information more effectively."

—*Risa Lavizzo-Mourey*

"Consider this: I can go to Antarctica and get cash from an ATM without a glitch, but should I fall ill during my travels, a hospital there could not access my medical records or know what medications I am on."

—*Nathan Deal*

As we have traveled across the country discussing physician burnout, we hear all kinds of concerns. Topics that crop up include the interference of the federal government, litigation threats, tone-deaf administrators, greedy insurance companies, and more. But by far the single-most commonly referenced "new stressor" is the electronic medical record (EMR). No other entity seems capable of raising such ire and invective amongst our colleagues.

To be fair, some physicians seem to have made friends with the EMR. Many are enamored with the technology and the multitude of ways that it can be employed in the care of their patients. Those who embrace EMR systems tend to be younger, having been raised in a digital universe.

With the simple flash of fingers across the keyboard, they seem to be able to access function-alities that many of us had no idea existed. However, this is not solely a generational issue. We know many highly computer-savvy people of all ages who deplore the EMR.

Those of us who are stressed by such systems seem to feel double-crossed. We were told the EMR was to be our salvation—technology that would save the healthcare industry billions of dollars and contribute to far better efficiency, quality, and patient safety. We were told it would free us from our bonds of documentation and liberate us to spend the maximum amount of time with our patients. We were told many things. Yet, according to both our anecdotal findings and accumulating empirical research, it seems that most physicians believe that the promises have yet to be fulfilled.

So many providers we have interviewed can tell long and detailed tales of the nonsensical lan-guage, algorithms, and work-arounds that must be employed to wring any sense of functionality out of their own systems. What is more, many are infuriated that the various electronic systems within their own medical centers do not intercommunicate (the general medical record system and the radiological imaging system, for example). And, of course, there is little or no electronic communication with EMR systems at other healthcare systems.

How do you feel about the electronic medical record? Has needing to interface with a computer screen driven a wedge between you and your patients? Have you found that it adds hours to the workday? Has it resulted in your having to bring home one to three hours of charting every night—and if so, is this negatively impacting your quality of life? Recent research showed that the more medical record work done after hours, the lower the self-reported satisfaction with work/life balance in physicians.[1]

Does the EMR allow and encourage excessive electronic access to you (for patients, nurses, technicians, clerical support, administrators, regulators, etc.)—heaping further workload onto your already-bursting-at-the-seams day? Do you sense that the EMR was designed for effi-cient billing and record keeping but not necessarily improved patient care? Do you feel that it encourages extraneous and nonsensical, if not blatantly inaccurate, copy-and-paste notation—even from yourself? Does your EMR system seem to be at times purposefully obfuscating and impenetrable? Have you ever simply lost it with your system, delaminating after reaching one too many fields to fill in, or one too many automated warnings about drug interactions?

If you answered yes to many of these questions, you are not alone. These feelings and concerns are ubiquitous amongst your colleagues. To more than a handful, the EMR is the single biggest evil in the world of medicine since bloodletting.

Yet, as with most storms that wreak havoc on our lives, when we shift our perspective a little, the proverbial silver lining usually reveals itself. The EMR is certainly not all bad. It has already solved many problems that used to plague our industry, and as the "bugs" get worked out, it will surely solve many more. We simply need to learn how to make the most of the EMR as it exists now and look ahead to a brighter future.

Here are a few questions for you to contemplate and discuss with your peers, friends, families, mentors, or perhaps a therapist. Please see www.studergroup.com/thriving-physician for more questions.

Consider and Discuss

- Design the ideal EMR. What functionalities will it feature? How will it be employed to improve patient care? What components of an EMR system are a must? How will your ideal EMR system differ from the system you currently use?

- Is it possible the EMR has become an easy scapegoat for some of your free-floating frustrations and anxieties about the healthcare world and its future? Could this be because the EMR is inanimate? How could you begin to see the EMR as an ally rather than a foe?

- Have you closed your mind to the "good" aspects of the EMR? List the functions that the EMR has improved in your practice or that contribute to better patient care.

- How might you learn how best to use your system? Who on your team or center excels at the use of the EMR? Can you learn from them? Are there other expert resources available to you?

Building Resilience

Okay, we get it. The EMR is thus far falling well short of its promise, far short of your expectations. It needs to do better. The concerns of those who must employ it out there on the front lines must be heard and acted upon. But as with all unpleasant interfaces within your harried medical life, we encourage you to ask, *what is the 10 percent of this challenge that I own, or that I can affect for the better?*

Clearly the EMR is here to stay. It is far better for your sanity and peace of mind to find creative and constructive ways to cope with it. Here are a few suggestions.

Rethink and reframe. In so many ways, the EMR is a godsend. Some of us can remember the days of paper charts, lab slips, EKGs, and celluloid radiographic films. In a clinic of 40-50 patients, maybe 10 of them came with fully intact records. Countless hours would be spent tracking down missing radiographs or sections of charts. Often, entire charts went missing. Consultant notes could be indecipherable due to the miserable handwriting of the average provider. Lab results may have been delayed for weeks due to misfiling or lost printouts. Now, with the click of a few keys, it all unfolds before you upon your screen—on your desktop, laptop, notepad, or even your phone. And acquisition of results from various radiological studies and lab tests are near instantaneous. It is a miracle of modern technology. Embrace it—you are lucky enough to live in an era where it is the norm!

Find meaning. Perhaps it is because we are accustomed to such user-friendly interfaces with the digital world these days (via our phones, our houses, our cars) that the EMR seems a bit too Byzantine in its functionality. But healthcare is a uniquely complex organism. A single patient can be infinitely complex in his or her care and needs (biological, medical, financial, legal, etc.). It will take decades to perfect a unified electronic system that will work seamlessly throughout all medical settings for all patient needs.

Don't believe for a minute that the major digital think tanks would not love to solve this riddle—there is too much money riding on it not to be so. For now, though, it is as if we were all mandated to take an unrefined "pill," one that holds great promise, but is in its earliest of stages of development. Only through experiencing and reporting the "side effects" will we refine the pill to the point that it reaches its greatest potential. Likewise, we are part of a process—frankly, a revolutionary process and one that will indeed bring better care to millions. But it is in its earliest stages and will throw up challenges. Tolerating your frustrations and seeking optimal ways to interface with these systems will contribute greatly to a whole new and wonderful level of patient care.

Embrace your new ally. One way or the other, these systems are here to stay. It does no good here to "chafe at the bit." Rather, we all need to chill a bit and recognize the EMR as an ally, a brilliant, multidimensional, and powerful ally at that. We need to invest some time upfront and learn the nuances of our specific systems so that we can truly employ them with maximum efficiency. Believe it or not, it is doable—just watch how facile our youngest colleagues are at it! Also, take heart that physician frustration with EMR systems is being widely recognized, and greater and greater effort is being made to streamline and make more user-friendly their functionalities. Perhaps it won't be long before you find the EMR as an indispensable colleague… perhaps even a friend.

In the meantime:

- Learn to love your technological support. Most medical centers have armies of technological support personnel. Don't hate them because they hail from a younger generation, and they speak a totally different language, and their fingers fly across the keyboard affecting unimaginable functionalities in your system. Use them, learn from them, have them on speed-dial!
- Learn from friends. If the "techies" are just too much for you to handle, seek out those in your center who are facile at the EMR. Buy them lunch and have them show you all their tricks.
- Write down the tricks and shortcuts you learn from others. Shown ten, you will remember only one and will become very frustrated.
- Engage your patient positively. Never complain to a patient about any aspect of the care you are providing—that includes the EMR! You are setting your own mindset in the negative, not to mention the patient's. Frame the EMR positively while asking for tolerance. Say something like, "Forgive me for typing. I want to capture the important details about your care, so we'll have a permanent record."
- At some point, completely detach from the computer—physically move away from the EMR and toward your patient. Make solid eye contact and ask an open-ended question. Let them speak for a while with your full attention. When you summarize the visit for the patient or have important information to impart, do so directly, face to face, not from behind the computer.
- Learn the shortcuts. This is critical. They do exist—even in your broke-down old system! Most systems are chock-full of shortcuts that can relieve you from so much misery. They can turn notation into super-fast exercises rather than supreme time sumps.

- Refresh. The systems are perpetually being upgraded. Learn the new functionalities and nuances of your system. Periodically check in with the experts on new timesavers.

- Don't take the work home. This is poisonous. Try to finish your charting concurrently with your visits or shortly thereafter. If you are having to complete your charting every night at home, there is a real breakdown going on. Most likely, you can learn EMR efficiencies that will obviate the need most of the time. If this is truly not the case, your work setting is dysfunctional and needs thoughtful and constructive addressing with your leadership. Discuss with your colleagues—are they in the same boat? When addressing system-wide dysfunction, there is strength in numbers.

- Insist on limited lines of communication. Many EMR systems have multiple communication lines for patients, administrators, providers, coders, etc. These are heaped onto your existing email addresses, social media platforms, phones, texting services, and more. Too much access to you can have toxic effects. Seek to limit access to a handful of mechanisms. Insist that others will simply not be answered. Again, discuss with your colleagues—see if you can come to a group consensus on what is appropriate access to the typical provider and stick with it.

CHAPTER TWENTY-SEVEN

Hello, My Name Is Inigo Montoya…

—From the movie *The Princess Bride*

Managing the Patients' Families' Expectations

"When everything goes to hell, the people who stand by you without flinching—they are your family."
—*Jim Butcher*

"But grief makes a monster out of us sometimes…and sometimes you say and do things to the people you love that you can't forgive yourself for."
—*Melina Marchetta*

In medicine, not only are you tasked with attending to the needs and wants of your "customers" (the patients), you are also quite often called upon to attend to the concerns and demands of their families (and close friends). Often your patients may be confused, or very young, or debilitated, or incapacitated. Under such circumstances, great amounts of discourse regarding their care must be conducted with their family members. Even when patients have full possession of their cognitive faculties, they may be overwhelmed and call for familial reinforcements. And even when patients are fully capable of interfacing with caregivers, family members may be invited, or may insert themselves, into the proceedings.

The stresses of illness and its attendant medical care can precipitate new, problematic family dynamics and/or magnify chronic, unresolved family issues. Many families are remarkably ill equipped to manage the disruption that comes with hospitalization or illness of one of their members. Families vary tremendously in their levels of sophistication and poise when facing the medical system. We have watched families tear apart and literally come to blows over granting permission for various medical interventions.

The appalling weight of potential downstream guilt is omnipresent. Loved ones grapple with thoughts like, *If I allow the surgeons to do this, mom may die, or she may survive only in a vegetative state. If I don't let them, she may die or be left in a vegetative state.* Despite intense counseling that there are no wrong answers in dealing with so many medical conditions, the specter of guilt cannot be shaken.

Another form of guilt is also frequently in play. Family members will torture themselves over what they might have done to save their loved one from his or her current state: *If only I had noticed her leaning to the side earlier. If only I had taken the keys from her after she had been drinking. If only I had insisted on taking him to the doctor when his chest pains first started,* and so on.

Furthermore, families face a barrage of other emotions when a loved one sustains a major injury/disorder. Fear of loss and grief are screaming at them every moment. Unfamiliarity and discomfort with the medical world and its navigation are nearly guaranteed. Ignorance of the scientific principles behind their loved one's illness is almost universal. Frustration, principally with the disease but also with the medical system, and its providers, is understandably common.

Somewhere along the line, unless miraculous improvements occur in their loved one, anger rears its head. It comes in many flavors: anger at the disease, at the uncertainty, at the byzantine nature of the healthcare system, at the slowness in the making of a diagnosis, or at the multiple small human errors in care (that to the worried family member seem massive and unforgivable).

This is where you, the physician, enter the fray. For the family, the world is coming to its end. But for you, this is one of ten significantly ill patients on whom you are checking (as rapidly as possible) this morning, before you head off to other duties. What is more, a room full of family members without question represents a time sump—time that you do not have. The family needs hours of soothing, comforting, and educating that you simply cannot provide.

One of our colleagues felt so pressed for time in his daily administrations that he would actively avoid patient families—not out of hard-heartedness, disrespect, or disdain, but out of fear of falling hopelessly behind. He would purposefully round in the early morning, before visiting hours. When approaching various ICUs, he would take back staircases to circumvent waiting rooms that so often bristled with anxious family members.

To make matters worse, you are often "set up" for conflict. Supporting personnel (nurses, therapists, aides, etc.) and often physicians from other specialties defer family members' questions and verbalized concerns to you. You are hailed to the patient's bedside. You yourself may still be awaiting further clarification and adjudication about plans for the patient from other physicians. The family demands enlightenment. You are not comfortable conveying much information. The fuse is lit, and all too often you are caught in the explosion.

A medical resident we know infuriated a family by entering a patient's room and checking on his progress through the night. The family expected an update on the patient's condition (including a yet-to-be-delineated liver biopsy diagnosis and definitive information on an array of unstable medical co-morbidities). The resident explained that she could not provide all the details they desired but would get back to them as soon as she could. The family saw red. They filed a protracted formal complaint against the resident, including a demand for her firing.

What is more, family members are often afflicted with profound cognitive and psychomotor shock when confronted with major injury or disease in a loved one. Their capacity to process often very sophisticated medical concepts and engage in multi-step decision-making is severely degraded. Thus, the cornerstone of meaningful human interaction—communication—is compromised. Repeated and extended counseling sessions are needed to fully effect understanding between the providers and the family members, and the physician simply does not have the time (and may not have the expertise) to provide such.

Here are a few questions for you to contemplate and discuss with your peers, friends, families, mentors, or perhaps a therapist. Please see www.studergroup.com/thriving-physician for more questions.

Consider and Discuss

- Have you ever been on the receiving end of a difficult family discussion about a loved one's health management? If so, what did you experience? And what did you learn from that experience that affects how you deal with families today? How often do you apply these lessons?

- Though families differ greatly, what are common underlying needs of many families?

- What are some methods that might help to put family members more at ease when discussing critical features of patient care (e.g., what is the best environment, sit or stand, identify a spokesperson for the family, go with support)?

- What do you do best when handling patients' families? Where are your opportunities for improvement?

Building Resilience

Interaction with patient families is unavoidable (and should not be avoided), particularly in the setting of critical illness. This will take time and emotional energy. Rather than view families as an anchor, enlist them as **allies** in the care of your patients. They can reinforce your efforts in educating the patient, as well as help assure his or her adherence to your treatment plans. They can tremendously bolster your patient's trust in you. They can help soothe your patient's fears and grief. They can often act as supplemental nurses and therapists.

Beyond this, families can be a major source of daily uplifts. Most are quick to warm to physicians who are upfront and honest, who spend time to teach, and who address them with civility and empathy. Many will be grateful for your time and effort for a lifetime. Many show incomprehensible grace in the face of great grief and/or calamity. They truly can be a source of restored meaning, inspiration, and even faith in days full of aggravation.

One of our neurology colleagues remarked that he keeps a drawer full of thank-you letters in his office—many of which are deeply moving. The majority came from family members of patients who died while under his care (patients who suffered from devastating strokes, ALS, Alzheimer's disease, etc.). He insists he did nothing spectacular for the patients, but he treated the patients and their families with patience and respect, and took the time to answer questions, teach, and soothe.

- Consider family members your "additional" patients. They are indeed significantly affected by their loved ones' illnesses and are ailing. Often they are ravaged as much or more by the patients' ailments than the patients themselves. Many patients eventually come to peace with their lots, whereas family members are often left devastated. By expanding your scope of care to the surrounding family (and close friends), you are greatly extending your "healing" influence far beyond a handful of people a day.

- Consider family members as future PR agents. Happy family members can be some of the most powerful proponents out there for you, your team, and your practice. The diaspora of family members with positive and even loving attitudes about you can extend far and wide.

On our busy inpatient neurosurgery service, we ran into significant family disaffection. We simply could not get to families at times other than the very early morning, or on the run between operations. We were barraged daily with nursing calls about upset family members craving contact and information. Formalized complaints were routine. We therefore developed and deployed a "hospitalist neurosurgeon" system. We dedicated one or two faculty surgeons to perform nothing but inpatient duties each week. This included daily walking rounds, timed to catch family members during visiting hours. The rounding surgeon spent as much time as necessary with each patient and family. Almost immediately, complaints dropped to near zero, as did distressed nursing calls.

- Seek efficiency in addressing family members of the critically ill when you are pressed for time (as you always are!). Here are a few suggestions to help manage this component:

- Try to gather as many family members at a time when addressing critical issues so you don't end up having to repeat the same information over and over again.
- Ask for a family spokesperson or two who can relay critical information to the rest of the family.
- Set specific times to meet with family members, so the greatest number can be already assembled when you come to speak with them. Enlist your nurses and other support staff to help you make the necessary connections.
- Include your support team in discussions so they can reinforce what you have said.

CHAPTER TWENTY-EIGHT

Madness…Madness…

—Major Clipton, *The Bridge on the River Kwai*

Dealing With Mayhem and Tragedy

"Why do we laugh at such terrible things? Because comedy is often the sarcastic realization of inescapable tragedy."

—*Bryant McGill*

"When sorrows come, they come not single spies,
But in Battalions."

—*William Shakespeare,* Hamlet

Many physicians are routinely exposed to a startling array of human tragedy and random mayhem. Examples might include:

- The innocent bystander shot in the head in gang violence
- The teenager dying from acute meningitis
- The 20-year-old with traumatic quadriplegia from a motor vehicle accident
- The 50-year-old father with pancreatic cancer
- The 4-year-old child with neuroblastoma who will face years of chemotherapy
- The premature infant who succumbs to respiratory failure
- The family badly burned in a house fire
- The young boy in sickle cell crisis

- The farmer whose arms are mangled in a machinery accident
- The depressed mother of three who jumped off a building

And so on...

The simple fact is that many patients present to the medical system in big trouble. The front lines of care, today's tertiary care hospitals, often resemble a war zone—and it might be you who is out there at the "sharp end of the spear." At many institutions, it is not uncommon for a physician to be called upon to evaluate five or more seriously injured or ill emergency room patients at a time.

You may be one of the early responders to a "trauma alert" and, thus, hear the recounting of the stupefying details behind a major trauma. You may participate in the initial injury survey and witness the gruesome carnage of multiple trauma. Furthermore, you may be the first on the team to interface with the shocked families and friends of the critically ill/injured and have to impart horrific news and details to them.

The incoming tragedies are relentless and seem to concentrate in the middle of the night. There is no regulator, and on some nights there may be no breaks.

> On the night previous to the writing of this chapter of the book, our on-call resident admitted three patients who were acutely quadriplegic from injury, three patients with severe closed-head injuries (all of whom went on to die), three patients with devastating intra-cranial hemorrhages, one patient with a gunshot wound to the head, and two patients with newly diagnosed malignant brain tumors.

This ferocity in exposure to tragedy and mayhem assaults even the most jaded of psyches. The only human experience that could approximate it for many would be war.

The exposure need not be quite this dramatic for the effects to be the same. All hospital-based physicians routinely witness the full gamut of injury to the organs and systems of their specialty. Ophthalmologists see traumatic enucleations, horrible infections, progressive blindness, etc. Neurologists diagnose Lou Gehrig's disease, a death sentence for the patient, and multiple sclerosis with all its attendant worries and disabling progression. Hospitalists contend with rows of patients in multi-system failure (many of whom will die or never make it out of a nursing home). Otolaryngologists wrestle with invasive and disfiguring head and neck cancers, orthopedic surgeons with exploded pelvises and horrifically contorted limbs.

Thus, almost regardless of your specialty, you are reminded with striking frequency that the human body is far more frail and vulnerable than the casual observer out in the "real world" might suppose. The course of so many lives are inexorably altered by the medical events that you routinely witness. With enough exposure, your world view begins to distort. You see the tragedy, mayhem, and sadness of the hospital as the real world, and the outside world of joy and health as a fantasy. You "normalize" the deviant experience of being in the hospital and start to view the outside world as being abnormal and undesirable.

> *On surveying residents, many noted that when they ventured out into the "real world" and witnessed happy, healthy people enjoying life, they would frequently be overcome by a pervasive sense of doom—that they would someday see these happy people again, all beaten up or desperately ill, in the hospital trauma bays and ICUs.*

And you are the rare physician if you do not give occasional pause for thought to the cosmic roulette wheel of fate, and to the notion that you inhabit a spot on that wheel. Personal vulnerability is constantly in your face. Somewhere echoing in the back alleys of everyone's mind has to be the thought, *that could easily be me on that stretcher*. Probably even more profound and heart-wrenching is the terrible notion, *that could easily be my loved one on that stretcher*.

As a physician, you may have to hear story after explicit story of horrific accidents, witness mangled limbs and bodies and faces and heads, cradle babies in your arms who will never awaken, tell families that nothing can be done to save their mothers, explain to grieving families that their 19-year-old sons will never walk again, tell young husbands that their wives have metastatic breast cancer, tell parents that their daughters are in severe respiratory distress. You cannot experience this on a regular basis and not be changed. You cannot go through years of this and not have a dramatically shaken view of the world, of humanity, of God. Vicarious traumatization, crisis of faith, compassion fatigue, burnout, and frank depression lurk behind every corner of a busy modern American medical center.

Here are a few questions for you to contemplate and discuss with your peers, friends, families, mentors, or perhaps a therapist. Please see www.studergroup.com/thriving-physician for more questions.

Consider and Discuss

- Do you think that it is necessary to become more distant, jaded, cynical, and/or nihilistic in order to survive the vicarious trauma to which you are exposed? How can you avoid this?

- How are your survival strategies learned from your work affecting your relationships outside of work and your general view of the world?

- Where are the rays of light amongst the carnage that you witness?

- Who on the outside "gets it"? Whom can you confide in?

- Do you ruminate about the tragedies you witness? Do they wake you up or keep you awake at night? Do you have related nightmares?

> *On surveying tertiary care physicians across the country, many admitted to relatively routine nightmares about their experiences at work. Many experienced sleep paralysis (new or at increased rates since beginning their medical career), and others experienced regular night terrors (several per month since beginning their medical careers).*

Building Resilience

There is no simple solution here. As discussed above, you cannot participate in healthcare at a modern American medical center and not be challenged and changed by the experience. Some will be more impervious than others, but no one will come through unscathed. Recognize that all sorts of complex feelings will surface as you witness the inconceivable carnage. It is best to acknowledge the sickening sense of randomness and vulnerability that it engenders rather than bury the feelings.

- Be willing to discuss your feelings and responses to what you have witnessed. This can be with trusted colleagues, family members, or friends.

- In debriefing with others, avoid blow-by-blow recounting of the events and move on to your responses to them: "I could not help but think of our own child today when I treated this young boy for injuries from an accident"; "I am deeply religious but I find myself questioning the benevolence of God when I witness good people being so horribly injured"; "I felt so helpless today when we were losing this patient in a cardiac code."

- Don't shy away from offering solace. Sometimes a simple, "I am sorry you had to experience that trauma alert—I heard it was dreadful," can go a very long way. We have found that such gestures, combined with a warm hand on the shoulder, are remarkably soothing and restorative. The great thing is, giving solace can be a remarkably soothing and restorative act for the giver as well as the receiver!

- Don't shy away from receiving solace. This can be particularly effective when coming from colleagues who truly "get" what you are going through.

- Work to create a culture where caring about your colleagues' emotional state is the norm.

- Beware of gallows humor. Some of it may offer a necessary release of tension or a protective mechanism against an erosive sense of personal vulnerability, but too much tips the scales into nihilism and going numb to the suffering of others.

- Beware of denigrating the patients or implying that they brought their tragedies onto themselves. ("Yes, she was horribly injured, but she was drunk!!" or "Yes, he has multiple brain abscesses, but he shoots up with dirty needles.") This is also a mechanism of fending off learned helplessness when facing the arbitrary nature of mayhem, but it drives a "humanity wedge" between you and your patients.

- Learn the signs of your own emotional depletion: Detachment, panic, cynicism, anger, sadness, tension, diminished cognition, rumination, frustration, nervousness, fatigue, sleep loss, agitation, inertia, and many other manifestations are possible.

- Listen to your body when it tells you that you need a break. Small breaks of calm meditation, a little sunshine and fresh air, a slowly sipped and savored cup of coffee, a phone call home or to a friend can all go a long way.

- Intersperse extended breaks into your work schedule—days or weeks off—particularly if you work in super-high acuity settings. Try to use this time to participate in activities that are particularly restorative for you and your loved ones. Avoid drama and instead seek joy and serenity. This sounds trite; however, disengaging from the hospital world of mayhem and tragedy often takes some upfront energy, something that will feel in short supply when you first break out. Try not to slump into a semi-coma on the couch. Collect positive experiences that you can carry back into the hospital and recall during your short sanity breaks.

- Maintain and strengthen your connection with your close relations. Watch for the tendency to pull away. Drifting away from those you care about the most is the antithesis of what you need. Seek out these people and actively invest time and effort in the relationship. Take interest in their world and their experiences. Share experiences. Refrain from the temptation to compare their work and life stressors with yours (and trivialize theirs). This helps no one and makes your loved ones feel less valued. And they will eventually be less likely to want to engage and share with you.

- Collect uplifts. A recurrent theme in resilience-building is the collection of daily uplifts. Believe it or not, even in the bleakest of medical circumstances, the potential for uplifts abound. You may not be able to save or cure a patient, but you sure can offer them comfort and caring. And you can do the same for their friends and families. They need your emotional and psychological support, and in so giving, you have fulfilled a sacred role of the physician—to offer comfort to the suffering. A few moments of humanity can generate a lifetime of gratitude. Soak this up. Acknowledge to yourself that you acted as a good doctor despite the wretchedness of the situation. Celebrate that you were an island of calm, competence, and kindness in a maelstrom of calamity.

CHAPTER TWENTY-NINE

Now I Am Become Death, the Destroyer of Worlds

—J. Robert Oppenheimer quoting from the *Bhagavad Gita*

Your Unrelenting Relationship With Death

"He that cuts off twenty years of life
Cuts off so many years of fearing death."

—*William Shakespeare,* Julius Caesar

"Golden lads and girls all must,
As chimney-sweepers, come to dust."

—*William Shakespeare,* Cymbeline

The physician's interface with death, and all that flows from it, could fill many tomes and never exhaust the subject. But let's be brief here and simply touch upon a few key components.

To most people in today's American society, death is essentially an abstraction. Their exposure to the real thing is rare and random. It in no way resembles the daily interface with death so often seen throughout the history of mankind. For most, it is the stuff of fantasy video games and cheap teenage thriller movies—where there is none of its wrenching emotional and meta-physical impact. The young and middle aged live in a society almost completely cleansed of the piercing reality of death and the despondency it can so readily engender.

Of course, many have had some passing exposure—the loss of a beloved but ancient and failing grandparent, or the automobile death of someone they vaguely knew in high school. But beyond this, death carries so little of its overbearing omnipresence, its stark inevitability, its stunning sting, its hollowing invasiveness, and its unfaltering finality. It is more a tale of a far-off land, or a nightmare from which one can always awaken into the safe embrace of modern life.

For you, however, death is an undeniable reality. Every day, you and you colleagues have the opportunity to interact with patients who die, who are rapidly cascading toward death, or who have come into profound risk of imminent or protracted death. And those who die hail from every age group: babies, children, teenagers, young adults, the middle aged, and, of course, the aged. Many were in fine health until their sudden demise.

Death is omnipresent in modern tertiary hospitals. It is a constant, only varying in the sheer number of unfortunate souls who "shuffle off their mortal coils" in any given week.

> *Residents interviewed across the country relate that no one they know outside of medicine can relate to their experience with death. They feel that others cannot possibly "get it." Most of their friends have zero exposure to death, whilst they exist in a modern-day charnel house.*

Exposure to so much death and dying is seldom given much consideration in our medical schools, residencies, and professional gatherings. We make very little allowance for our own response to the phenomenon. Even if we care for dying patients daily and absorb the surrounding tension and fear of both patients and families, we seldom take time—or are given permission—to process or mourn.

In addition to our feelings of loss and grief for our patients, persistent exposure to the uncompromising finality of death must incite in most of us a sense of personal mortality and a concern about the vulnerability of our loved ones. Several physicians with young sons and daughters that we have interviewed note the profound impact the death of a child has on them. They cannot help but worry and ruminate about the welfare of their own children. Others relate gnawing and persistent anxiety about the welfare of their life partners.

We are sure that such sentiments give you pause for thought at least now and then. Surrender to these worries, however, can result in psychic contraction and paralysis. To avoid this quagmire of existential pain, if you are like many of your colleagues, you "whistle past the graveyard," denying the enveloping and oppressive reality. Resultant "gallows" humor and seeming callousness is so very rife among us all, and it can easily be misinterpreted by any outsider as cruelty and sociopathy.

Unremitting exposure to death also carries a real risk of learned helplessness: the mentality that, no matter what is done, death will continue its macabre saunter through the ICUs and trauma bays. Going numb, nihilism, cynicism, and irreverence come next.

> *Neurosurgery residents we have interviewed admit to the development of a profound insensitivity to death—a numbness and an impenetrability, born out of the incessant exposure. They rarely think about it, yet they feel its presence, always lurking, always ready to "drop in." They report that the constant exposure tends to trivialize all other problems encountered. They have a hard time hearing residents from other services talk about bad outcomes, often thinking, "Well, at least your patient isn't dead." They have an equally difficult time hearing loved ones and friends lamenting about work or home issues, often thinking, "Well, at least no one has died on you today!"*

To further complicate matters, you may have to come to grips with the fact that you played a role in hastening or even causing a patient's death, either unwittingly or intentionally (DNR, withdrawal of care, "comfort care," etc.). You can easily succumb to an oppressive weight of guilt and culpability. You can be haunted by the refrain: "If only I were better at this, I might have been able to save this person."

Few come into medicine truly prepared for this "dance with death." The finality of it all can challenge every tenet of your faith and world view. You will not be able to skate by this one. One way or another, the impact of such an intimate relationship with the grim reaper will insinuate itself into your thoughts or dreams.

Here are a few questions for you to contemplate and discuss with your peers, friends, families, mentors, or perhaps a therapist. Please see www.studergroup.com/thriving-physician for more questions.

Consider and Discuss

- With whom do you talk about death?

- How has so much exposure to death affected your spirituality?

- Did anything in life or in school prepare you for the sheer volume of death that you have encountered in medicine? What helped?

- How do you feel when a patient wishes to speak with you about death? What is behind those feelings?

- How often do you worry about the vulnerability of your loved ones and friends? Do you tell them about this? What can you do to alleviate some of the anxiety?

- If you were to impart your best advice, what would you tell medical students, residents, and physicians about dealing with patient deaths?

Building Resilience

As with mayhem and random tragedy, there is no easy solution here. Recommendations from the last section may help but, with respect to death, you must first accept that your intimate association with it is an anomaly in today's society. Few of your acquaintances and loved ones outside of the hospital can relate. But it is not their fault, and you should not trivialize their world and concerns. Next, you must acknowledge that your exposure to death impacts you no matter how much you suppress it, and no matter how little you think it does. Too much exposure is toxic without some form of relief.

Critical to diffusing death's impact is **debriefing**—discussing with others your exposure to death. This does not mean a blow-by-blow recounting of each death, but rather exploring your reactions to the process. Were you sad, frightened, angry, relieved, numb? Did it affect you physiologically? Did it invade your peaceful moments, including time with your loved ones and your sleep? What complex thoughts and feelings did it engender? Clearly colleagues are a great sounding board because they share your experience, but don't discount your friends and loved ones. They will be less jaded, nihilistic, and irreverent, and may be better equipped to plumb some of the deeper ramifications with you.

Read treatises on the subject. Others before you have contemplated this. Try writing your own thoughts down. Sometimes it helps simply to release your emotions out onto a piece of paper. Furthermore, don't discount clergy or psychologists/psychiatrists. This interface with death is "big league" stuff and may at times warrant professional help.

We believe that "disenfranchised grieving" is a nearly universal part of the psychosocial "underbelly" of life as a physician. It is healthy to grieve. This may not be readily acknowledged or fostered by colleagues, family, or friends, but it should be. Whether or not you have had a close relationship with the deceased, their death will affect you. Throughout your career, develop and maintain rituals that allow you to honor patients who have died. Allotting yourself some moments of sadness and meditative or metaphysical thought is critical to healing. Burying these very primal responses to death will lead only to negative emotions bubbling up unpredictably and often in very maladaptive ways.

> One of our internal medicine colleagues recalled encountering a striking series of deaths over a very short period of time. He could not sleep the following weekend, so he watched a series of silly movies. During a scene from Field of Dreams, he found himself weeping uncontrollably. Eventually, he poured himself a tumbler of Irish whiskey to regain control of his emotions. He considered how the scene dealt with the passing of a father and a son's longing to have had more time with him. Our colleague realized that the scene had released the dam of emotions and related contemplations that had built up during the previous week's overwhelming exposure to death.

As a physician, encountering death is an anticipated, unavoidable part of your professional life. Here are a few further ways to try to cope.

- Have due compassion for yourself.
- Allow yourself to identify and express feelings about your witnessing of death and dying.
- Be supportive of your colleagues. Simple words of compassion can instantly normalize the pain for them (e.g., "I heard about your patient. So sorry. I've been there, too. This is difficult. If you want to talk about it, I am here."). Such words help soothe the existential reeling that comes with the experience and gives a colleague hope for a less painful future.

- Accept support back. Research has shown that support offered by peers in the wake of a patient's death helps to foster adjustment and resilience.
- Honor and remember fondly those who have died.
- Hug your loved ones.
- Sometimes, go ahead and cry at a silly movie.

CHAPTER THIRTY

My Kingdom for Some Dilaudid!

The World of Pain

"The greatest evil is physical pain."
—*Saint Augustine*

"The great art of life is sensation, to feel that we exist, even in pain."
—*Lord Byron*

No matter your specialty, it is almost a foregone conclusion that you will have to at least dabble in the world of pain. Pain is a ubiquitous and universal human experience, and to one degree or another, it is interwoven into almost every ailment that we face. Cancer, a twisted knee, volvulus, zoster, a broken jaw, heart attack, pulmonary embolism, arthritis, MS, a tooth abscess, migraines, pleural effusion, skin infection, and so much more, all involve to one degree or another a significant component of pain. Dealing with patients in pain, and with their concerned loved ones, will likely occupy a sizeable portion of your medical career.

Treatments for pain, both medical and surgical, are seldom universally successful or fulfilling. And people in pain do not necessarily make for the happiest and most grateful group of patients. Think about the last time you were in a lot of pain. Think of the discomfort of just making it to an appointment of any kind. Many pain patients grow accustomed to being bounced from one specialist to another, which they invariably perceive as being given "the runaround." So therefore many are frustrated, impatient, depressed, apathetic, or even angry and hostile.

You want so much to be able to help them, but often you cannot. This engenders a sense of failure and hopelessness that can be extraordinarily draining. You so often leave their exam rooms feeling totally empty.

The management of vast volumes of patients in pain can become overwhelming for any physician. The spine surgeon, the family practitioner, the orthopedist, the orthodontist, the podiatrist, the otolaryngologist, the neurologist, the gastroenterologist, and scores of others will all generate a growing list of unhappy pain patients even from the most motivated of clientele.

Furthermore, not all pain patients are well motivated or well intentioned. The psychosocial world of pain is vast and multi-dimensional. It is affected by mental illness, secondary gain, litigation, drug-seeking, depression and anxiety, medical co-morbidities, individual tolerance, and so much more.

Pain patients can be profoundly unhappy, demanding, and sometimes manipulative. They may call at all hours of the night and day with fantastic stories of narcotics bottles taken away by twisters or struck by lightning (both actual tales recalled by colleagues). Some may become out-and-out hostile.

> *Our neurosurgery practice receives several hundred narcotic-related phone calls every week, quite a few of which devolve into tantrums, invective, and overt threats.*

It takes a special physician to treat a high volume of patients in pain and maintain a sense of efficacy and humanity. The stark juxtaposition of remarkably stoic patients who should be complaining about their horrific cancer pain and the abject manipulative chicanery of some of your pain patients can be stupefying. It can lead to a warping of your impression of your fellow man. It can crystallize a sense of futility, cynicism, suspicion, and derision when dealing with all patients in pain. You run a serious risk of developing a very jaded and hard-hearted sense of the world.

Not very long ago, we (of the medical community) were chided, if not vilified, by "authorities"—the federal government and the media—for not covering patients' pain sufficiently. Now, with an epidemic of narcotic abuse ripping through our society, we are chided and vilified by the same entities for employing too many analgesics. The care of pain is therefore a bit of a minefield through which most physicians navigate with growing trepidation.

Here are a few questions for you to contemplate and discuss with your peers, friends, families, mentors, or perhaps a therapist. Please see www.studergroup.com/thriving-physician for more questions.

Consider and Discuss

- Have you ever been in severe pain? Have you ever been in unrelenting severe pain? What was the experience like? How did it affect your mood and your personality? How did you feel about those who were not able or did not choose to help you? How did you feel about those who actually did help you?

- What would it be like to be in so much pain that you could not hold down a job? What would you do to survive? What resources are out there to help? Are there any? How would you access them?

- When a patient keeps coming back to you, unresponsive to your administrations for their pain, what do you feel? What do you think? How quickly do you tire of the patient? How long can you be empathetic? Do they need to improve for you to remain engaged and compassionate?

- If a patient is not to come to you for relief of pain, where should he or she go?

Building Resilience

A major driver of the discomfort of dealing with pain patients is the feeling of lack of efficacy that they can engender in you; nothing you do seems to help.

- Recognize that the battle with pain is not an all-or-nothing affair.
- Focus on the complaint. Study it. Look for at least partial solutions.
- Remind the patient that some improvement is better than none and that a pain-free existence might be a tall order.
- Apprise yourself of pain-related resources in your region.

- Don't shy away from non-traditional methodologies. If a patient swears that an alternative treatment helped their pain, celebrate it with them. Anything that helps, helps!

- Remind yourself that the patient is the one with the problem. At the end of your interaction, you move to the next patient; they remain with the pain. Most times (but not always), you did not give them their pain. You are simply trying your best to help. Continue to try your best. If you can do that, your own discomfort will ease.

- Recognize that it can be rather difficult to be empathetic with pain patients, particularly chronic pain patients. You are not in their shoes; you are not experiencing what they are experiencing.

- Try to think of a time when you were in real pain or at least some discomfort. Magnify it and imagine it being prolonged and relentless.

- You may not want to offer up much in the way of narcotics, but you can offer understanding and compassion. For the patient who has become used to being brushed aside by so many practitioners, even this much will seem like a breath of fresh air.

- Try not to personalize your patient's venting. Give them a sympathetic ear—with ground rules. Draw the line at abusive behavior directed toward you or any on your team.

- Try to steer clear of internally dehumanizing or denigrating these patients. You went into medicine presumably because you liked people and wanted to help them. The reduction of human suffering is hopefully still a core driver in your day-to-day professional existence. Devaluing your patients will begin to eat at you. Remind yourself of the patient's humanity and their need for help and support. Be kind. Actively listen.

CHAPTER THIRTY-ONE

I Am Surrounded by Buffoons!

The Risks of a Holier-Than-Thou Attitude

"Never seem more learned than the people you are with. Wear your learning like a pocket watch and keep it hidden. Do not pull it out to count the hours but give the time when you are asked."

—*Philip Dormer Stanhope, 4th Earl of Chesterfield*

We sometimes fail to understand and fully appreciate the nuances of each other's specialties. From here it is easy to develop a "holier-than-thou" attitude. As you practice your specialty, you may quickly realize that you are one of the few providers in your institution who is truly adept at handling your chosen organ system when it goes awry. These capabilities certainly may inspire pride and a sense of bonding within your team, but it can go too far. When this occurs, it can become easy to overvalue what you know and undervalue others' unique competencies. This is a dangerous precedent, one that can lead to an intellectual arrogance signaled by your nonverbal judgments or overt slights.

It can be easy to slip into an attitude that you are the only one who is competent, dedicated, or hardworking in your hospital. Every time a provider from another specialty opines on "your" organ system, they may in your opinion prove to be laughably naive and on unsteady ground.

> *One of our endocrinology colleagues reported that she initially felt bemused by the hospitalists' consult requests about hormonal issues. They were routinely misdirected. Eventually, though, she became distrustful of any endocrinological assessment or intervention initiated by any other type of physician. When a provider from another specialty started to report their interpretation of a patient's hormonal status, she would find herself unintentionally tuning out.*

You are at risk of seeing yourself as a lone wolf within a dysfunctional ecosystem. You may come to view other healthcare workers with condescension. You may become prone to bouts of righteous indignation when other providers don't perform to your standards. Such emotions are difficult to completely hide, as cynicism and sarcasm bubble to the surface.

Other providers may thus come to see you as caustic and unpleasant and withdraw from your company. In turn, the sense of team diminishes. "Collaboration" and "integration" become platitudes that you utter to make system leadership happy but have no real role in your patient care. Care is delivered from specialty silos. You see your specialty as a fortress under siege rather than a member of a "league of nations." This not only compromises patient care, it precipitates a sense of isolation and loneliness.

Here are a few questions for you to contemplate and discuss with your peers, friends, families, mentors, or perhaps a therapist. Please see www.studergroup.com/thriving-physician for more questions.

Consider and Discuss

- How often do you feel a condescending attitude toward your coworkers? Why? Do they notice it? How does it feel when another specialist is condescending to you?

- How far does your righteous indignation go? Do you carry home unrealistic expectations for loved ones, friends, family members, acquaintances, workers, mechanics, store clerks, waiters, children, pets?

- Is it wrong to place a higher value on work/life balance than you do? How much sacrifice do we owe our patients? How much is enough?

- Can you learn from physicians in another specialty? Can you learn more about your specialty from a physician in another specialty?

Building Resilience

No one can know everything in medicine. High-level modern healthcare depends on integration and collaboration between multiple teams of physician specialists, as well as with allied healthcare workers. Everyone plays a part in the ultimate outcome of the patient.

One of the great joys of the modern team approach to care is that you can learn so much by simply speaking with your coworkers from other specialties. You may even learn more about your own specialty. Various specialties and various individuals come at medical problems from different angles and vantage points. They afford you the opportunity to "see the familiar in unfamiliar ways." This may be a huge asset when tackling a perplexing problem. Besides, it makes medicine less lonely and less anxiety-provoking. It can also be a catalyst for the blossoming of friendships and the impetus for collaboration in research and education efforts.

- Envision taking on a patient with multiple organ systems in trouble. Envision taking on everything by yourself. Envision the patient slipping further and further downhill. How does it make you feel? Are your palms sweating yet?
- Now picture a consultant from another specialty seeing the patient. He is curt and sullen, and he admonishes you for the timing and the nature of the consult. He writes a few unhelpful lines in the patient's chart, "signs off," and disappears. How do you feel now? What do you think about this consultant?
- Now imagine another physician from yet another specialty entering the fray. Imagine that she is friendly, complimentary, helpful, and even jovial. Imagine her helping you get things under control. Imagine her returning as often as you need, and her being complimentary to your work. Imagine the patient making a nice recovery. How do you feel now? We would venture a lot better than earlier. How do you feel about your colleague? We would bet pretty grateful and beholding.

Which scenario do you choose to represent how you practice? We encourage you to commit yourself to being the specialist in your field whom everyone loves to see come in on a case—the physician who is always helpful and complimentary and thus is always deeply appreciated.

CHAPTER THIRTY-TWO

Where Is the Love?

On-the-Job Isolation and Loneliness

"We are all sentenced to solitary confinement inside our own skins, for life."
—*Tennessee Williams*

"Loneliness is proof that your innate search for connection is intact."
—*Martha Beck*

Being a physician can be a remarkably lonely undertaking. This may seem counterintuitive when one considers how many people you interact with in a day. But let's face it: You are on the run from the minute you start the day until its belated end. All interactions are hurried and all are "business oriented." There is no socialization, as your task list is endless and any interaction only slows you down.

What is more, in this modern era, you may interact with a computer for more hours a day than you do with other human beings. True connection or psychological intimacy takes time, time that is nowhere to be found in your crammed schedule. So, you end up eschewing interaction in order to avoid starting what you don't have time to finish.

Then there is an element of experiential isolation, the sense that no one "gets" what your world is like. No one else seems to be working as hard, or is on the run so frenetically, or is pulled in so many directions, or is so sleep-deprived and chronically tired. This perception is not entirely far-fetched. Few other professions do compare in work demands, hours on the run, and duty hours through the night.

If you are still a resident, the hierarchy is such that the chasm between you and a resident just one year senior to you can seem unbridgeable. Furthermore, all the residents in a program are so rushed with their own duties that there is almost no opportunity to congregate and share experiences. Residents of the same training level are often assigned to other institutions or sub-specialty services, thus offering little opportunity to interact with "fellow travelers."

It is not so very different for practicing physicians. Most see few of their partners in a typical week. There is an old adage that "If you really like someone, don't go into practice with them— you will never see them."

On call, you are truly out there all alone. The night fills with calls from people you do not know, to see patients you have never previously met. You materialize in various locations, but only long enough to address the problem at hand and then move on to the next. The long, empty, fluores-cent-lit hallways seem to stretch out further and further like a Hollywood-depicted nightmare, your worn-down shoes plodding along endless echoing institutionally grey tiled floors.

On the home front, things don't get much better. Engaging in intimate relationships takes physical, psychological, and emotional energy. Your fatigue is often construed as disinterest. This tends to alienate significant others, friends, and family. And, when you do emerge from the strange psychosocial "twilight zone" of your professional world to engage in social interactions with "normal people," you no longer share much in common with non-physician others.

> *On interviewing residents across the country, most reported profound bouts of loneliness and social isolation. Loneliness was one of the greatest sourc-es for job dissatisfaction. Many of our residents reported significant difficul-ty relating to acquaintances. They felt that no one seemed to comprehend what they were going through. They reported particular dismay over com-ments from family members like, "Oh, honey, things can't be as bad as you say!" They reported feeling annoyed when others (family members, friends, or non-neurosurgical residents) compared the hardships of their work to their own.*

Thus, you can go through your days often feeling very alone in a sea of humanity. The hospital takes on the feel of a prison with you locked away in solitary confinement. This is no frivolous matter. Research with young adults has shown that loneliness is a significant impediment to resilience and well-being, and a risk factor for a multitude of physical, behavioral, and emotional maladies.[1,2]

Here are a few questions for you to contemplate and discuss with your peers, friends, families, mentors, or perhaps a therapist. Please see www.studergroup.com/thriving-physician for more questions.

Consider and Discuss

- When do you feel most connected with other physicians? When do you feel the least connected?

- Who in your personal life do you think best understands what your world is like? How often do you interact with this person?

- Do you isolate yourself from others at home and at work with electronic media? How can you separate yourself from such activities?

- What do you know about the personal lives (backgrounds, interests, hobbies, etc.) of those with whom you work intimately on a daily basis? Colleagues? Nurses? Technicians? Support staff?

- With whom might you spend a few minutes engaging in conversation and fellowship when you are on call?

Building Resilience

Oh boy, this is a big one, and probably due more than this short contemplation. One of the critical components to remaining resilient is meaningful connection with others. And in your job, it can be so difficult. It is extraordinary how isolated and lonely you can feel when you are surrounded by so many people. But the potential for connection is there, and it is critical that you find it and put energy into maintaining it. If you do, you will find that the energy invested is paid back double (in new positive psychic energy). No, you cannot stop and chat with everyone you interact with in a workday—you would never get anything done. But you can find islands of connection throughout the hospital.

- Focus on the places you frequent the most, and for the greatest amounts of time. Think about how you usually function in these settings: all business, rushed, harried, all dials set to maximum efficiency. The people around you could be mannequins or robots for as much as you recognize their humanity.

- When at one of your "home bases," pause for a moment and open your eyes and ears. Make eye contact. Truly greet those you see most often. Don't keep things totally superficial. Begin to learn a little about their lives, thoughts, and ambitions. Ask questions and listen and register the answers. Follow up the next time you come by: "How are your daughter's applications to college coming?" or "How did the big football game go for your son last weekend?"

- Be more than a blur to those you work around. People are friendlier, more anxious to connect, and more willing to share than you would imagine. A few short exchanges can open up vast areas of fascinating discussions, anecdotes, and channels of exploration that can truly enrich your life (thoughts, philosophies, experiences, books read, music appreciated, places to visit, restaurants to try, TV shows to watch, etc.). Plus, you may build some deep and rewarding new friendships.

> *A friend of ours, Pat, is particularly skilled at this phenomenon. He can rapidly find great interest in virtually anyone he meets. Within seconds of interacting with anyone—from any walk of life—he can enter into an in-depth discussion about an unusual hobby, a new political philosophy, a strategy for home improvement, the best car engine on the market, and much more. People warm to him immediately and greet him like a long-lost family member the next time they see him. Through this he is a fountain of information—on almost anything—and is recognized and loved throughout his community.*

- Use some of Pat's tricks: Make a real effort to engage with people. Give them undivided attention and ask probing questions. Listen intently to, and process, the answers while demonstrating a body language of true focused engagement (eye contact, leaning in, raising of eyebrows, appropriate nodding, etc.). What you are doing is validating the existence of the person with whom you are engaged, no matter their social or professional standing. You are offering palpable respect. This engenders tremendous engagement and appreciation. You may not be adept at this sort of interaction, but you can develop these skills. The payoff is a deconstruction of the environment that fosters your feelings of isolation and loneliness. Try it out, at work and out in the real world. You will be amazed and gratified at the response. But a warning here: The interest must be sincere. Walking up to a ward nurse and saying, "It has been a cold week, eh?" while you are checking social media on your phone won't cut it.

- At home, you also must seek connection and engagement. While it is healthy to share components of your day with loved ones, they don't want a blow-by-blow recounting of the indignities that you suffered or how unhelpful everyone is around you. A steady barrage of this sort of exchange will drive them away and further your isolation. Rather, recounting of the day should be a shared activity. Exchange some positives and negatives and, most importantly, their effects on you. Ask for the same from your loved ones in return. At some point, let the events of the day go and turn to synergies, plans, new ideas, fresh thoughts, and things to anticipate together.

CHAPTER THIRTY-THREE

I Am Lost in the Twilight Zone!

Distorted World View and Arrested Social Development

"A man walks down the street. It's a street in a strange world. Maybe it's the third world. Maybe it's his first time around. He doesn't speak the language. He holds no currency. He is a foreign man."

—*Paul Simon*

"I can't go back to yesterday because I was a different person then."

—*Lewis Carroll*

As a resident or a physician in practice, you are totally immersed in a foreign world. You seldom see the light of day. Your work schedule is ridiculous, and the daily demands are insatiable. Unimaginable multi-tasking is the norm. Your work environment consists of color-sapping fluorescent lighting, cries and moans, shrill electronic tones, and often horrible and/or surreal sights. Your emotional environment is filled with mortality, sadness, tragedy, bad news, loneliness, hostility, and performance anxiety. Inescapably your world view begins to distort—a world that is a vast deviation from what most others encounter becomes your norm.

To put it in psychological terms, you have "normalized a deviant experience." What to the casual observer would be perceived as a strange and disturbing existence has become your day-to-day. Most would seek to escape such an environment if given the opportunity. Yet you are submerged in it for the grand majority of the waking day. It becomes your norm, and the world on the outside becomes the outlier.

When you do venture out into the "real world," you will notice how unusual it all feels because it is not what you have grown accustomed to. You may feel unmoored because you are not surrounded by the sick, the dying, the critically injured, the sad, the hurting, the terrified. The people around you will move at a different pace from what you are used to. Likely, their thought-processing, decision-making, and actions will seem deliberately and intolerably slow to you. You are used to the supercharged, multi-tasked environment of the modern medical center. Further, no one will seem in "crisis mode." People will seem inordinately happy and carefree. Believe it or not, this may feel very strange and disturbing to you.

When you do break free of the hospital, you will also be prone to feeling rather interpersonally stunted. Your medical immersion is so total that you know of little else. When you attend a social event, you may not know what to say or even how to act. After all, you are not up on the news, recent movies, or the latest music. You are not much savvier about social media than are your much older colleagues. You have no sense of what is "in" and what is fashionable. You feel that your humor is not at all in sync with others.

In interviews with residents across the country, universal themes of distortion of perception of the "real world" came to the fore.

Residents expressed surprise at the number of people outside "who did not look deathly ill," at the great numbers of people who were smiling and seemed happy, at how frequently they saw people who looked healthy and who were engaging in healthy activities.

They also noted a different pace of life. People appeared unhurried and unharried; they seemed to be enjoying leisurely meals and ambling walks in the park. One resident marveled, "Unlike in the hospital, most of the people I encountered were friendly, kind, and polite."

Residents reported feeling quite uncomfortable in these surroundings. In an unexpected twist, several reported a longing to be back in the hospital environment after a period of time "out there."

What is more, when engaged in conversation with the denizens of the real world, many residents noted other difficulties and discomforts. They felt that, compared to what they routinely witnessed in the hospital, the problems discussed with "laymen" were superficial and trivial. They expressed a sense of surrealism to conversations that seemed so important, but that did not relate to life-and-death circumstances.

They found that they had trouble appreciating the humor of the outsiders, and that outsiders had little appreciation for their own "gallows" humor.

They found it bizarre that so many people seemed preoccupied with world events and/or politics.

Universally, they were incredulous at what others thought was "hard work."

Residents also reported a discomforting sense of potential doom when interacting with the seemingly happy and healthy. This was born of experiences in their medical worlds that suggested that disaster was always lurking just around the next corner, for anyone and everyone. Intruding into their streams of consciousness were haunting thoughts that these happy people could be the next broken bodies to be wheeled into their trauma bays.

For many physicians, immersion in the world of medicine leaves them culturally marginalized. Their lack of cultural integration strengthens their sense of isolation and loneliness, and their discomfort with social situations fosters reclusive behaviors. Their natural response is to retreat to the environment that they feel most comfortable in, that of their work!

This can quickly become a reverberating circuit. Constant exposure to the deviant environment distorts your mental map of the world and makes you uncomfortable and more than a little socially incompetent outside of its walls. Therefore, you seek to spend even more time in the hospital, making you even more uncomfortable with the outside world. We know many physicians who absolutely prefer to remain cloistered within the medical center rather than venture out into normal society. They find every excuse to stay locked away, and, of course, the medical world offers infinite opportunities to keep occupied within it.

> *Many of the providers we have interviewed note a growing reticence to venturing out into social situations. They report that classic "cocktail parties" have become anathema. When thrust into such situations, they are happy only upon leaving or when another team member shows up and they can talk about work.*

Here are a few questions for you to contemplate and discuss with your peers, friends, families, mentors, or perhaps a therapist. Please see www.studergroup.com/thriving-physician for more questions.

Consider and Discuss

- Do you feel an increasing distance between your work world and the outside world? How? Why? Which is more real to you?

- Do people close to you feel like you have changed since you became a physician? In what ways? Do you agree? How do you think you have changed?

- How many people really want to hear the nitty-gritty details of your medical world? Should it be more? How should they respond?

- Do you try to keep abreast of current events, current fashions, current music, current entertainment? If so, how? If not, how might you?

Building Resilience

It is important to resist totally normalizing the hospital environment. It is not normal at all. Accepting it as your new normal could make you "tone deaf" to the myriad of stressors that you encounter. Horrible, tragic things are still horrible and tragic. Unrecognized, they will take their toll.

An environment of bright, cheerful places filled with happy, healthy people is the "real world" and is a critical source for energy restoration. You must get out of the hospital.

- Engage with your fellow healthy humans, revel in their happiness, appreciate their health, and enjoy their friendliness.
- Don't let your circle of friends and acquaintances contract down to your teammates. Open yourself up to conversation—no matter how trivial it is compared to your professional life. Regular interaction with a circle of happy, healthy friends recharges your batteries.
- Make some time to experience what is going on out there. Poke your head up out of the foxhole and read some newspapers and magazines. Watch a couple of TV series or catch a ball game or two. Familiarize yourself with the celebrities of the minute, the star athletes, the actors and actresses. Learn a bit about your local landmarks and geography. Dabble in a little political discourse. This is the currency of normal, happy exchanges between acquaintances and casual friends.
- Keep it light at first. As your friendships deepen, you can occasionally tackle the hard stuff. But going to a party and reminding everyone that you "cannot imagine a loving God after the stuff you saw this week" will not get you invited back. Speak the language of common social intercourse and enjoy turning your serious mind off for a while.
- Try to bring a bit of "normal" into your work environment. Engage in friendly chatter now and then; ask coworkers about their lives outside of the hospital; share interests and hobbies; talk about sports or books or movies. By doing so, the disparity between your work world and the outside world diminishes, and the transition between the two seems less abrupt.

CHAPTER THIRTY-FOUR

You First!

The Impact of Fear

"I understand that fear is my friend, but not always. Never turn your back on fear. It should always be in front of you, like a thing that might have to be killed."
—*Hunter S. Thompson*

"Things done well and with a care, exempt themselves from fear."
—*William Shakespeare*, Henry VIII

Fear is an underestimated component of practicing medicine. It lurks about the back allies of most physicians' minds. This is not necessarily always a bad thing. Fear of causing harm manifests positively as respect for the delicacy and fragility of the human body and its various systems. It reinforces sensitivity and care in all medical and surgical interventions.

If you are an internist, you should have a lot of respect for, and perhaps a modicum of fear of, the powerful medications you prescribe to your patients. Just listen to a pharmacological commercial on TV now and then. Remember that list of 50 horrific complications they tag on to every ending: "This medication may cause itching, swelling, temporary or permanent blindness, eyes dropping out of their sockets, chest discomfort, chest pain, heart attack, congestive heart failure, sudden cessation of heart beat, sudden heart combustion and implosion, etc."

If you are a surgeon, you should fear damaging tissues, or whole organ systems, or the entire organism (the patient) in your surgical manipulations. All tissues should be handled with the utmost of care.

When you pause to think about it, you—and all physicians—will realize that you can hurt patients in so many ways: through patient management oversights, lack of vigilance, overt errors, lack of relevant knowledge, from receiving misinformation, being unclear in your directions, some unforeseen reaction or complication, or from just plain-old bad luck. And the patients aren't getting easier. So many today are riddled with multiple serious co-morbidities. The margin for error is often razor-thin.

In addition to harming patients, physicians deal with a myriad of other fears. Consider the fear of embarrassment. Physicians are raised in a culture of embarrassment. Medical educators certainly use this one as a major motivating tool in medical education (think of the Socratic method as applied in medical training). But this fear goes on for the remainder of a career.

For example, most physicians feel markedly embarrassed when they make errors in judgment or diagnosis, or cause some form of complication, or sustain a poor patient outcome. So many physicians aspire to perfection in all their administrations that anything short precipitates this profound embarrassment. They fear being perceived as being stupid, lazy, careless, ill-prepared, or inadequate. They fear losing the respect of their colleagues or even failing in their practices. Thus, fear of professional embarrassment can literally alter a physician's approach to a patient's problem.

In our interviews of residents, most reported that the fear of embarrassment was one of their strongest nemeses. Yet, it was also one of their strongest drivers—to read, study, and practice. Few believed that the somewhat acerbic Socratic educational method employed by so many programs should be toned down. Nonetheless most reported physiological stress responses to the "classic" residency teaching methodologies (grand rounds, escalating questions, mock boards, oral quizzing, scientific reviews, etc.). Interestingly, many reported that another major fear was that of disappointing the faculty members with their academic, research, and operative performances.

Sometimes the embarrassment you feel is totally internal. We bet that you, like so many physicians, suffer, to one degree or another, from an "imposter syndrome." That is, you have a hard time wrapping your head around the fact that you are a mature adult with a lofty and venerated position in society. You cannot imagine that you—yes, you—are caring for those who really need you and all your expertise. Are you truly that competent? Or are you just a "poser"? Wrestling with this question can be terrifying. Yet, those who don't can drift very easily into narcissism and unjustified self-belief.

Add to this list the modern hospital fear of "write-ups"; of doing poorly on various accrediting exams; of administrative admonitions for EMR-charting and behavioral inadequacies; of angering patients, families, and nurses; of being rated poorly online; and of the ever-lurking litigation lawyers.

When you face formal complaints about your level of care or your behavior, the risks of psychosocial distress soar. A recent study reported that physicians who received complaints about their care were more than twice as likely to report moderate/severe depression, anxiety, thoughts of self-harm, and suicidal ideation than those who did not receive care complaints.[1] Some days the modern medical center feels like a minefield, and, whether you recognize it or not, you respond physiologically with fear (and sympathetic overdrive).

Here are a few questions for you to contemplate and discuss with your peers, friends, families, mentors, or perhaps a therapist. Please see www.studergroup.com/thriving-physician for more questions.

Consider and Discuss

- Discuss a time when someone in the workplace complained about you. Putting aside your outrage, what other feelings did this stir in you? How does fear of this happening again affect you? How do you feel when you walk onto a floor where you know people have complained about you?

- How often are you embarrassed at work? Is this useful in your education/development? What embarrasses you most at work?

- What situations elicit a sense of fear or the physiological response of fear in you? Hurting patients? Complications? Embarrassment? Angry patients? Angry families? Risk of write-ups? Risk of litigation? Risk of recognizing your own shortcomings? Risk of mistakes? Giving bad news? Having to discipline someone? Fear of being an "imposter" as a practicing physician?

Building Resilience

This is where we get to tell you to put on your big boy or girl pants and get out there and attend to those in need. The reality, as discussed above, is that fear in the practice of medicine can be healthy. In a limited dose, it keeps you alert, sharp, and focused. It pushes away lassitude and a lackadaisical attitude. It reinforces a sober respect for the frailty of the human body and its tissues and a respect for the risks of all interventions. We don't advocate the elimination of fear from the practice of medicine. Rather, we advocate its control.

Some disease and patient predicaments call on you to be very brave. And bravery means pushing forward and doing your job or duty despite the fear. Someone has to make the tough decisions, to take the risks, or to deliver the bad news.

> One of our colleagues muses: "You know, we can't always do that much for our patients. But we sure as heck should have the guts to speak to them and their families openly and honestly. When you think of it, we are paid a lot of money to be brave enough to at least tell the truth about things."

If fear is taking the "front seat" in your work, you need to find ways to bring it under control.

- Try to identify what exactly is driving the fear. Is the fear generated by serious patient situations where the risks of your decision-making and/or interventions are high? If so, focus on your physiological response to the situation rather than all the potential pitfalls of it. Relaxation techniques and methods to reduce the physiological response are of great use. Exercises in breathing, meditation, mindfulness, focusing, and calming may all be useful.
- Step away from an anxiety-provoking situation for a few moments, if you can. Try to turn off the mental chatter and rumination about the situation. Envision a positive process and outcome.
- Forgive yourself for some fear: "It is okay to be uptight about this case; the risks are high."

- Seek strength in numbers. When facing a high-risk situation, ask colleagues to help you or offer advice. The addition of just one more "player" can significantly reduce the level of anxiety for you as opposed to taking it on all alone.

- If your fear is more related to personal anxieties revolving around embarrassment, admonitions, or self-doubt, consider the source. Does it truly need to be responded to with fear and/or anxiety? Are patients going to be harmed? Are you going to come to physical harm? Does it at all matter in the grand scale of the universe that you felt embarrassed for a few moments? Will people remember this and think less of you for time immemorial? Can you laugh at this with others someday? How does it compare with the indignities that your colleagues have suffered?

- Forget perfection. Many of our anxieties revolve around ego and a misguided belief in perfection. Forgive yourself for your lack of perfection. Strive for excellence instead of perfection and recognize that shortfalls will arise now and then.

- Remember, you are the real deal! As for being an imposter, forget it! You are no imposter! You were among the smartest of the smart throughout your academic career. You are well trained, and you have committed yourself throughout your life to excellence. If you are not fit to do this job, then who else is?

CHAPTER THIRTY-FIVE

I Believe, I Believe; It's Silly, But I Believe

—Natalie Wood in *Miracle on 34th Street*

Crisis of Faith

"Religion can be both good and bad; it is spirituality that counts."
—Pat Buckley

"To me, spirituality means 'no matter what.' One stays on the path, one commits to love, one does one's work; one follows one's dream; one shares, tries not to judge, no matter what."
—Yehuda Berg

It may well be true that there are no atheists in foxholes, and there are probably very few in the middle of a complex and dangerous medical intervention that is going poorly. Most physicians have been known to offer up prayers, or other invocations to a higher power, at various critical points in their administration of care to their patients, no matter their predisposition to organized religion. Many enter medicine with very definite theological underpinnings. Some remain very devout throughout their careers. Others may place their faith less in theological entities, but in more humanistic-oriented conceptualizations. One way or another, however, one's faith is certain to be rocked and tested by the discipline.

In life, there is a staggering array of ways in which the good and the innocent can be subjected to unimaginable suffering: the child with leukemia undergoing chemotherapy and bone marrow transplantation; the pregnant mother hit by a drunk driver sustaining severe multiple trauma; the sweet family man with pancreatic cancer undergoing palliative procedures; the loving grandmother devastated by a massive stroke, hooked up to all sorts of tubes and devices in an ICU. Every specialty has its share of mind-numbing tragedies and horror shows, and you get a front row seat to it all.

Beyond this you may also get to witness the savage sequelae of human depravity, stupidity, cruelty, and ignorance—particularly if you work in an emergency room or trauma center.

There is no way that anyone's mental map of the way the world should be is not warped and potentially fractured by their exposure to life in a busy university medical center. This may be particularly true if one enters the field with a strong faith in a loving God and/or an orderly universe. In the hospital, life is distilled down to its most base and its most primal. The sense that tragedy and suffering is arbitrary—perhaps even gratuitous—and that the universe is a cold, unyielding, and cruel place can be inescapable. You will invariably question what it all means and how it could be this way. Wherever you rest your faith, be warned: Your whole system of beliefs *will* be shaken to its core.

Here are a few questions for you to contemplate and discuss with your peers, friends, families, mentors, or perhaps a therapist. Please see www.studergroup.com/thriving-physician for more questions.

Consider and Discuss

- What were you taught, and what have you believed about the following?
  - There is deep order and reason to life.
  - The good and the hardworking will be rewarded.
  - Dedication and persistence matter.
  - Everyone deserves a "second chance."
  - Despite hard knocks, everyone has some goodness inside.
  - Right usually rules over wrong.
- How have your experiences in medicine impacted these and other deep beliefs?
- What are your sources of spirituality?

- How often do you discuss your spirituality with others? Who is most open to such discussions?

- How do you feel when patients and their families ask you to pray with them?

Building Resilience

"Spiritual fitness" is actually a cornerstone of resilience. Considerable evidence exists that higher levels of spirituality correlate with greater well-being, less mental illness, less substance abuse, more stable marriages, and better performance across settings.[1]

As have designers of resilience training for the U.S. military, we emphasize that spiritual fitness need not be theological or religion-based. Rather, it refers to a belief system about what is "right" in interacting with your fellow human beings. In discussing spirituality, we refer to one's notions about "truth, self-knowledge, right action, and purpose in life; living by a code that is rooted in belonging to, and serving, something the individual believes in *that is larger than the self.*"[2]

- Realize that a busy medical center is a distillery of human misery. Suffering, tragedy, and mayhem are concentrated to surreal levels. When in the hospital, you are not in the real world. The real world is infused with so much more light and joy and beauty and happiness, and it is critical to get out into it whenever possible, to experience it.

- Open up your senses within the hospital. You will witness extraordinary examples of humanity, kindness, compassion, sympathy, connection, and grace. Grace, in particular. The very same patients who should be the most bitter and angry about their lots are so often those who exhibit preternatural levels of grace. Let your faith in humanity be recharged by embracing those who suffer their disorders with such grace and optimism.

- Escape the charnel house atmosphere of the hospital when you can and drink in the feast for the senses that so often exists just a few hundred yards away. (That's easy for us to say—the Blue Ridge Mountains are right outside our back door!)

- Soak in the camaraderie of your colleagues and admire their fortitude, empathy, and humor in the face of the horrors they witness with you.

- Remember that your work *is* sacred. That giving of yourself to help others is what spirituality is all about. That you are acting in good faith when you do all you can to help a patient, and to anticipate that your administrations will indeed be helpful to the patient. That you, your colleagues, and your patients belong to a most special congregation.

- Try this exercise: For a week, write down acts of grace, kindness, bravery, dedication, brilliance, unsolicited helpfulness, compassion, sweetness, selflessness, and honor that you witness at work. Read these back to yourself in the evening. We would bet that the examples are myriad and that the effect will be soothing and inspirational.

Remember, it is okay to share your thoughts about the larger implications of all that you encounter. But realize that colleagues, family, and friends likely have at least a somewhat different and very personal system of beliefs. Try not to proselytize. Listen carefully to the way others process their experiences. Look for common ground in spirituality. Seek positive approaches rather than abject nihilism.

CHAPTER THIRTY-SIX

Ah, What's the Use?

The Scourge of Nihilism

"Life's but a walking shadow, a poor player, that struts and frets his hour upon the stage, and then is heard no more; it is a tale told by an idiot, full of sound and fury, signifying nothing."

—*William Shakespeare*, Macbeth

"A cynic can chill and dishearten with a single word."

—*Ralph Waldo Emerson*

Everyone who works in the medical field—regardless of role or specialty—knows the dark and discouraging truth: We are engaged in a struggle against an enemy that will never capitulate. Every day, we fight a retreating action against the unstoppable forces of aging, disease, and death.

We see firsthand seemingly meaningless levels of suffering and despair. We work so hard to save each and every patient, and yet many outcomes are far from optimal. Sometimes our "saves" even leave patients in states that most would consider worse than death. In the midst of such futility, it's no wonder so many physicians come to adopt a nihilistic worldview.

Fueling this nihilism is the fact that suffering befalls people regardless of age, sex, ethnicity, or creed. Think of the 40-year-old with diffusely metastatic breast cancer, the 20-year-old in irreversible coma from a motor vehicle accident, the premature baby with multiple organ failure and severe brain damage. Then there are those who seem unwilling or unable to help themselves: the unrepentant smoker with lung cancer, the drug addict with bacterial endocarditis, the morbidly obese man with diabetes and secondary end-stage renal disease.

You are likely exposed daily to the massive medical expenditures (of money and resources) on hosts of individuals who will never regain a sense of self, or others who will never contribute in any way to their own health. It's no wonder you begin to question the point of it all. All your "blood, sweat, toil, and tears"—to what end?

> *We repaired a very complex constellation of cervical fractures in a man who sustained his injuries drag racing in the city streets. On his way home from the hospital, he was goaded into riding "shotgun" in another race. His car rolled over in the race, and he shattered his construct, necessitating a "front and back" cervical-thoracic fusion and several months in a halo vest.*

No matter how inherently gracious and kind you may be when you start your life as a physician, experiences like these will make you vulnerable to becoming cynical and nihilistic. On bad days, you may count on one hand the patients you feel you truly helped, and perhaps dozens for whom you had little or no impact. The seeming futility of so many of your interventions can blur your focus on the deeper meaning of your work, and without meaning, your resilience will erode.

Here are a few questions for you to contemplate and discuss with your peers, friends, families, mentors, or perhaps a therapist. Please see www.studergroup.com/thriving-physician for more questions.

Consider and Discuss

- What aspects of your world view (your beliefs about life, its "rules," and the nature of people) have shifted as your medical career has progressed?

- What positive lessons are you learning from some of the most painful experiences you are having?

- How badly does work-related nihilism and cynicism spill over into your thoughts and behaviors at home? How does it affect how you view stories depicted in books and movies? How does it affect your view of news and world events? How does it affect your view of medical interventions for friends and family members?

- What can be gained from the care of the hopelessly ill?

Building Resilience

Two principal antidotes to burnout are *meaning* and *engagement*. The more you feel like your work has meaning and is making a difference, the more you will feel engaged. And engagement at work—when you are involved, connected with your coworkers, and excited to "dig in" on the challenging problems of the day—is supremely energizing. It leaves you in a good mood at the end of the day. The better your mood upon arriving home, the happier you will be with your personal life and relationships. The happier you are in your personal life, the better prepared you will be to engage during your next stint of work. This is the *resilience cycle*: positive engagement and its corresponding positive moods, cyclically perpetuating each other.

Abject nihilism and its wretched sibling, unbridled cynicism, will suck the meaning right out of your work and set off a negative cascade that leads to disenchantment, detachment, misery, and burnout. Resist the very real temptation to see the negative in all events and situations. Beware that cynicism, while sometimes funny, fans the fires of disengagement and trivializes what you are doing.

Some suggestions (and we know we are getting a bit preachy here):

- Focus on the person behind all the extenuating circumstances. Tell yourself, *So what if this man is a drug addict. He is a human being and he needs my help.* Search for the dignity and the humanity in everyone. If you are having trouble divining it, provide the dignity and humanity yourself.
- Remember, everyone is stripped of much of their dignity and humanity the minute they enter your medical center. Treat everyone with respect. Introduce yourself. Listen to them. Maintain eye contact. Touch. Explain. Solicit their concerns. You will be surprised at how many people blossom, and how much easier it becomes to fully engage.
- Stay humble. Recognize that despite your very hard work, you have long ridden a wave of *cosmic good luck.* You are brilliant, conversant, insightful, and industrious. Odds are you came from a loving household filled with books, and that people sacrificed much to get you to where and who you are. Many patients you will encounter never had even a shred

of such luck. The cosmic roulette wheel may have dealt them bad genes, bad parents, bad perinatal care, bad nutrition, bad environments, bad education, and more. Maybe meeting you will be the first bit of luck they have experienced in their entire lives.

• When caring for the extreme elderly, imagine the patient as the person they once were: younger and more vibrant. Ask the family for some help in this. Solicit some details on the person lying there in the bed. Think of how you would want to be perceived and treated if you were in a similar situation and offer a good dose of dignity and humanity. We so often have so little to really offer in medicine, particularly to the very sick and elderly. Consider making your intervention one of respect, kindness, interest, and engagement.

• Recognize that every interface with a sick patient is an opportunity to sharpen your clinical acumen. No matter how hopeless the situation, no matter how bizarre or ridiculous the surrounding circumstances, every interaction is practice for the care of everyone else who follows. Learning from every encounter creates a path that will transport you from being a good doctor to being a great doctor. Those difficult-to-deal-with patients offer you a master's class in great patient care.

• Reap the benefits. Giving it your all for every patient, treating every patient with dignity and respect, staying positive and hopeful won't go unnoticed. Nurses see it. Attendants see it. Families definitely see it. Your reputation for being a truly caring physician will spread like wildfire. It will do more for expanding your practice than any PR department could dream of.

CHAPTER THIRTY-SEVEN

Everybody's Got a Little Larceny Operating in Them

—Bing Crosby in *White Christmas*

Ethical Challenges in "Everyday" Medicine

"Relativity applies to physics, not ethics."
—Albert Einstein

"The only tyrant I accept in this world is the 'still small voice' within."
—Mahatma Gandhi

Thankfully, virtually all medical schools nowadays include some level of ethics training in their curricula. Until recently, this was seldom the case. Often, such sessions explore several highly contrived scenarios designed to challenge the fundamental underpinnings of societal ethical constructs: "A pregnant, developmentally delayed hemophiliac is crossing the international time line when someone must decide which of her four fetuses should be harvested in a mother-threatening procedure for experimental brain implants to save the lives of the other three..." and so on.

The ethical challenges in your busy practice tend to be a bit more mundane, but they are protean and remarkably prevalent. Consider the following:

- For every diagnostic or therapeutic intervention a physician performs, there are other physicians "out there" who can perform it better. How does one reconcile moving ahead with the intervention while knowing this?

- Modern medical conceptualization of various diseases has become hyper-complex. Few patients will ever truly fully comprehend their disorders. How does one then establish true "informed consent" with a patient for a planned medical or surgical intervention?

- Many patients requiring acute medical/surgical intervention are not of ideal behavior or social background, often bringing trouble onto themselves. Do we inherently pass judgment on our patients regarding the worthiness for exceptional care? Does this ultimately affect their care?

- The indications for medical or surgical intervention in many disorders are rather "grey," yet the interventions can be very financially rewarding. How do we assure that we are always making our medical decisions in the *patient's* best interest?

- In the course of our medical careers, almost all of us will encounter physicians who are incompetent, or are malignant in personality and behavior, or are both. If such a surgeon lands on our team, or in our community, what is our obligation to assure that he or she will do no harm? What if they are simply not as good as you, or are simply average?

- A "shaken baby" has sustained severe diffuse brain injury. Prognosis for severe developmental delay is essentially certain. He will only ever function as a severe burden upon society. How aggressively should he be treated?

> *We sought to tally the ethical challenges of "everyday neurosurgery" in our practice over a month's time. We found that examples amassed so rapidly that we could not keep up with them.*

Challenges for the resident may even be more omnipresent. Consider the following examples specific to residents:

- If I ask the attending for help in this intervention, he will take it away from me. Isn't it okay if I take some risk and keep on going? I have to learn!

- Damn! I got a "wet tap" on this epidural. If I tell my attending, she will be upset. No one will know if the patient doesn't get a spinal headache.

- I am so tired of rewriting this journal article; perhaps if I took a few lines from this remote paper I found, the chief will finally be satisfied.

- The boss asked if I read up on this case last night. I meant to, but I fell asleep. Should I tell him "yes" and fudge it? If I tell him "no," he'll chastise me.
- Look at that family—all waiting for word on Mrs. Jones's tumor. I can't face them all weeping. Shall I tell them the tumor may need other treatment and let the oncologist give them the really bad news of its malignancy?
- Dr. Smith stinks at ERGDs, but he has a "bee in his bonnet" and wants to do a complex ERGD procedure on patient Garcia. He is probably going to do a crummy job. Do I keep my mouth shut and collect another "sticker" for the case? With whom could I discuss this? Would I get fired if I did? Who am I to judge?
- I smelled alcohol on Dr. Simonds's breath last night when he came in for that emergency shunt. Everything went fine. What should I do?

And so on…

Think also about the challenge for a faculty physician at a teaching hospital. The more autonomy this physician allows his or her residents, the faster they will become proficient in their specialty. Yet, the more autonomy the residents exercise, the greater the chance of complications for the patients. How much of a complex intervention should be performed by a resident? And for that matter, how much of the resident's role in a patient's care should be divulged to the patient?

The barrage of ethical quandaries can be near constant. Each one must be adjudicated by the physician according to his or her system of beliefs. Societal "norms" may help give direction but can also create significant internal conflict—the medical world is far from any "norm" that most people encounter. Physicians are often faced with "lesser of two evil" dilemmas. The ethicality of various decisions becomes much murkier for those who have minimal control of their lives and fear for their futures were they to "make waves" or fail in their "duties" too often (i.e., residents or junior practitioners). We believe that this constant hum of ethical decision-making often flies "under the radar," but creates moral distress that can erode resilience.

Here are a few questions for you to contemplate and discuss with your peers, friends, families, mentors, or perhaps a therapist. Please see www.studergroup.com/thriving-physician for more questions.

Consider and Discuss

- What lessons have you learned from times you have had competing values and had to decide a course of action that violated (at least to a degree) one of your values or beliefs about right and wrong?

- What do you think are the most basic principles of ethical medical care?

- How do you handle a situation where your ethical underpinnings come into direct conflict with your patient's (e.g., a pre-op patient who refuses a blood transfusion on religious grounds, parents who refuse to have their child immunized, etc.)?

- Are there others about you who clearly ascribe to a different set of ethical principles? If so, how might you reconcile this?

Building Resilience

There is much written about ethics in medicine and its classic ethical quandaries. Beauchamp and Childress identified four principal values that could be applied to a large swath of medical ethical issues.[1] These included the following: *Autonomy*: the right of the patient to choose their care/treatment; *Justice*: the equal availability of proper care to all; *Beneficence*: the expectation that the caregiver will seek to do what is best for the patient; and *Non-maleficence*: the expectation that the caregiver will seek to do no harm to the patient.

Multiple other tenets may also play into ethical considerations and quandaries, such as expectations of competence, societal responsibility, honesty, full divulgence of information, patient education, diligence, availability, respect, compassion, privacy, and more.

Ethical principles may offer you a foundation to build upon when facing particularly vexing quandaries, but they often don't hold all the answers. You and your colleagues are charged with finding the answers. Often the foundational principles can come into conflict with one another. It is perhaps best to approach this world first understanding your sense of ethical care. What principles are most important to you? Ideally, you might plumb why you hold onto these principles and how strongly you hold onto them.

- Be aware that everyone about you may not rest upon the exact same ethical underpinnings.

- Recognize that you are processing ethical decisions at a remarkably rapid pace.

- Recognize that at times you may need some time to stop and consider the decisions you are making.
- Try to be aware of decisions and interventions you make that challenge your ethical moorings.
- Be aware of your emotional and physiological responses. If you are feeling particularly stressed about a decision or action, consider which of your own ethical principles may be at risk.
- As with so many challenges to your resilience, a major source of decompression is open discourse and debriefing with trusted others. Colleagues will often be very helpful. A friend or family member may be even more so as they will offer a markedly different vantage point. Try to present the situation without coloring it with your own judgment.
- Be open to different viewpoints. Realize that over time most people's ethical principles shift and evolve. The real world has a way of softening the sharp edges. Realize there is no definitive authority. If you feel particularly confused, ambivalent, or affronted by a particularly sticky ethical quandary, most institutions have ethics boards that might help you find the way through the morass. Trusted clergy could be another valuable resource.

CHAPTER THIRTY-EIGHT

Winning Isn't Everything; It's the Only Thing!

—Vince Lombardi

Perpetual Peak Performance

"Peak performance in life isn't about succeeding all the time or even being happy all the time. It's often about compensating, adjusting, and doing the best you can with what you have right now."

—*Ken Ravizza*

"The temptation to quit will be greatest just before you are about to succeed."

—*Chinese proverb*

A baseball player is considered exceptional if he achieves a base hit once in every three times he is up to bat. But as a physician, you are expected to "hit a home run" every time you tend to a patient. You cannot have a "bad game" and certainly not a bad streak. Essentially every patient interaction is the World Series. Every diagnosis, every order, every examination, every test ordered, every intervention, every procedure is expected to be performed at near-perfection. This demand for excellence does not soften in the face of significant personal adversity—after a sleepless night on call, after a recent procedure gone horribly wrong, or after battling the flu all week. No matter the circumstances, you are expected to saddle up and perform.

Furthermore, you do not have the luxury of powering up to peak performance for just one "big game" and then cruising for the rest of the week or season. For most physicians, there are many, many "big games," every day and every week, not to mention tons of "night games" as well.

Essentially, you must find a way to activate the components of your highest level of performance—concentration, critical thinking, hyper-adaptable thinking, vigilance, calmness under fire, judgment, technical execution, and dexterity—hundreds to thousands of times a year, under any and all conditions.

If you are a resident facing these dynamics, the stakes are even higher. You are not armed with years of experience, thousands of cases under the belt, or hundreds of accumulated tricks of the trade and nuances. Instead, you are like a high school baseball player inserted into the last game of the World Series.

There are enumerable studies and books on how to elevate the star athlete to their peak performance for the "big game." Many of the measures described would likely dwindle in effectiveness if they had to be sustained for weeks, months, and years. Yet this is the world of every physician. Our society has established an expectation that its physicians function perfectly, at their utter peak performance, perpetually, under any circumstance. Failure to do so may result in hospital quality board reviews, safety committee evaluations, medical staff evaluations, and, of course, litigation.

Here are a few questions for you to contemplate and discuss with your peers, friends, families, mentors, or perhaps a therapist. Please see www.studergroup.com/thriving-physician for more questions.

Consider and Discuss

- Compare and contrast what it takes to sustain peak performance in an athletic endeavor to the performance demands you face in medicine.

- How exhausting is it for you to perform your specialty? What tires you out the most? Why?

- Who among your fellow residents and/or attending physicians seem the best at "ramping up" their peak performance? What are their secrets? Do you ever discuss this with them?

- What factors impact your peak performance? How can you alter their impact?

- If you are undergoing a medical intervention, what do you expect of your physician?

Building Resilience

You are called upon to perform at peak mental and physical levels all day long—day in, day out. Over the past few decades, much ground has been made with the preparation of athletes for peak performance in competition. Why could not the same approach be taken with physicians? Many peak performance resources are available. Some underlying principles, however, are fairly common to many:[1,2]

Positive Personality	Confidence	Motivation
Focus	Perceived Social Support	Concentration
Managing Emotions	Managing Anxiety	People Skills
Controlling Self-Talk	Setting Goals	Attitude
Using Mental Imagery to Prepare for Performance		

- Consider the relationship between anxiety and peak performance. Most texts acknowledge that there will be anxiety prior to competition and that most athletes enter an event somewhat on edge. The sympathetic arousal manifested somatically by increased heart rate, clammy hands, dry mouth, etc. may better prepare the athlete for physical peak performance. Too much anxiety, however, is crippling and leads to athletic hesitancy, clouded thought, over-thinking, and loss of focus and concentration.

- Be aware of your physiological response to the professional and interpersonal tasks of your day. Be on the lookout for a sympathetic overdrive.

- Practice managing your anxiety. Acknowledge that a degree of anxiety before a patient interaction and/or a procedure is natural and even potentially helpful (promotes vigilance, focus, attention). Practice relaxation, mindfulness, and breathing techniques to circumvent anxiety overload and its physiology.

- Consider the benefits of visualization. High performers across disciplines report that they regularly deploy mental visualization prior to every performance or competition. Elite skiers envision every gate of their upcoming race. Virtuoso musicians picture, hear, and feel every movement of the piece about to be played. Try constructing mental imagery for a positive and successful patient care scenario. Don't envision a disaster, but do incorporate "recovery" moves and decisions, anticipating some reasonable challenges to the "perfect" patient care progression.

- Consider the value of goal-setting. Athletes clearly define what they seek to accomplish in their competition and in their careers. These are called *outcome goals*. Likewise, many physicians motivate themselves with notions of the outcomes they are pursuing: an amazing patient interaction, the perfect surgery, the ICU patient being extubated, a month without complications, the happy patient leaving the hospital. Outcome goals have a twist, however; they may be subject to external forces that can greatly negatively affect the outcomes (e.g., caring for a patient with multiple severe co-morbidities). Outcome goals are seldom entirely in the hands of the individual performer and thus are subject to disappointing counter-outcomes and even abject disaster. This can lead to profound disappointment, helplessness, and disengagement.

- Consider focusing also on *performance goals*. These focus on specific aspects of your performance, ones that you can control—no matter the circumstances. Such goals give clear-cut targets for your energies and efforts. They thus can heighten focus and concentration and inspire commitment. Goals should be realistic and potentially within reach but should be somewhat of a stretch. Set goals that make you use your skills and push your limits. As you reach your goals, be willing to redefine and upgrade them.

- Sit down with a paper and pencil (or iPad) and outline some goals. If you are a resident, consider *performance goals* for rounds, presentations, exams, interactions, and for each patient interface. Create some *outcome goals* for procedures, interventions, rotations, PGY years, and careers. If you are a practicing physician, consider *performance goals* such as patients seen per clinic, timeliness of chart completion, journals read, papers written, committees joined, dinners with family, and activities with loved ones. *Outcome goals* could include physician ratings, successful procedures, thank-you notes, national presentations, papers accepted for publication, etc.

- Don't neglect the effects of imperfect outcomes on self-confidence. Neither physicians nor top athletes are perceived as coming up short in ego. However, the reality is quite different. Both groups are faced with frequent reality checks that come with less-than-perfect performances and utter failures. "I may not be quite as good as I think I am" is a haunting private refrain that every high performer has to learn to deal with. Explore and discuss the deflated self-confidence that comes when therapeutic interventions go poorly.

- Believe in yourself. How can you keep momentary setbacks from leading to diminished effort, diminished risk-taking, diminished perseverance, and more? How do champion athletes take the next final shot in a game after having missed a potential game-winner just days prior? They allow themselves to have "short memories." Champions are willing to get back into the fray. They believe in themselves and in their capabilities, skills, training, experience, intuition, and drive. This belief in self is critical to performing at your best. And why should it not apply to you? You have the intelligence, the training, the skills. Learn from mistakes, make the appropriate corrections, and then jettison the memory of the mistakes and gear up for your next challenge. Additional ways to approach:

- Review peak performance techniques used by athletes.
- Read some peak performance books.
- Consider engaging a peak performance expert to lead group discussions.

- Find a way to create breaks in the action. Truly give yourself a day off now and then. And during a busy workday, create five minutes of "space" here and there to calm down your physiology. Meditate, breathe, catch some sunlight.

CHAPTER THIRTY-NINE

My Work Is My Best Friend

The Decay of Close Relationships

"No man is an island,
Entire of itself,
Every man is a piece of the continent,
A part of the main..."

—John Donne

"When your father dies, say the Irish,
you lose your umbrella against bad weather...
When your father dies, say the Welsh,
you sink a foot deeper into the earth...
When your father dies, say the Russians,
he takes your childhood with him...
May you inherit his light, say the Armenians..."

—Diana Der-Hovanessian

Following your long workdays with few or no breaks, you return home drained and fatigued. The couch and the TV beckon. Connecting with others—even your closest of friends—feels like a monumental task. How can you be expected to find time and energy to link up with those important to you? And when you do, how do you make the connection interactive, positive, and intimate?

Many physicians simply don't. Sooner or later, they experience strained and deteriorating relationships with those they love. You are likely to fall into the same trap. You are likely to gradually withdraw, with predictable effects. Friends will complain that you are no longer available to "hang out." Extended family and parents will fret over drop-offs in communication. And, of course, spouses, life mates, and children will voice concern over your perpetual absence. In turn, you will feel increasing angst over perpetually abstaining from seeing your friends and loved ones. Nonetheless, you will find it harder and harder to make contact. If you do not curb this cycle, those same loved ones and friends will begin to withdraw from you.

As your stress mounts and social networks dwindle, you may become increasingly dependent on the few (if any) people who remain active in your life. If you are in a marriage or partnership, you may find that your significant other has essentially become your "caretaker," handling all household duties, constantly nurturing and soothing you, and putting you back together week after week.

Like many physicians, you may have taken a position in a region far from your original hometown, leaving you without built-in affiliations or easy access to close friends. Most relationships are new and must be nurtured and grown. And this, of course, takes energy—energy that you don't have. Your main "relationship" is with your work. Recent research showed that, compared to other U.S. workers, sevenfold more physicians work 60+ hours/week: 42 percent of physicians versus 6 percent of other U.S. workers.[1]

When your relationships are strained by your relentless stress and fatigue, everyone concerned suffers. Your life mate may experience their own isolation and loss of support. Remember, they too have likely moved far from home. If you are a parent, your mate will often live like a single parent, taking on all parental responsibilities, day-in and day-out—and do so without much community support.

> *In our recent survey, 89 percent of life mates of physicians stated that "as a family, we feel grossly misunderstood in our community," and that "neighbors seem to believe that we are living a stress-free life of a wealthy physician family."[2]*

The signs of failing personal relations stack up. Conversations become sparse. Flare-ups and frustrations become frequent. You become overwhelmed with guilt as you feel incapable of contributing to the relationship, yet continuing to take so much from it.

> *On surveying our own residents, all reported substantial decreases in contact with friends, relatives, and close relations. Only 12 percent reported routine continued contact with friends outside of the hospital. Only 12 percent reported continued close contact with their families. All reported a sense of sadness and guilt over their diminished contact. All residents involved in lasting relationships reported persistent strain between them and their significant others predicated on lack of time spent together, lack of shared activities, perpetual fatigue of the residents, and more. All reported increased numbers of "silly arguments" and "spats."*

Here are a few questions for you to contemplate and discuss with your peers, friends, families, mentors, or perhaps a therapist. Please see www.studergroup.com/thriving-physician for more questions.

Consider and Discuss

- Who would you interact with more if you could? What would you do with them? What would you talk about?

- How can you generate interest in other people's lives? What components of other people's lives interest you the most? What about your current life do you want your closest relations to know and understand?

- How often are you dismissive of other people's experiences because they are not as intense and critical as yours? Is this valid? How can you better validate their experiences in your own mind?

- When you come home at night, what is your status? Do you simply shut down? How much attention do you need? How much soothing do you need? How much attention and soothing do you offer to your significant other (if applicable)?

Building Resilience

No man (or woman) is an island. Sustaining positive contact with people important to you is a critical factor in sustaining your resilience. Each stressor discussed in this book can challenge your caring connections with loved ones. Burnout at work precipitates burnout at home and vice versa.

- Don't give in! Commit to connecting with those important to you. Resist the temptation to flop onto the couch at night. Be proactive with your relationships.

- If time is short, perhaps you could combine some activities. Ask a friend if he or she would like to go to the gym with you or go with you to the library to read while you catch up on your studies or go to the grocery store with you.

- Set up "dates" with your friends. Go out to dinner now and then; it doesn't have to strain your budget—a cheap burger joint is fine. Go for a walk in a park. See a movie. Work on a mutual hobby.

- Keep in touch with your extended family. You have your parents for only so long. It has been said that when your parents die, you lose your greatest fans. Cherish your time with them. Call them. Visit. Share with them your work—they will be fascinated and proud. Write them a letter of gratitude now and then. Send them plenty of pictures of you smiling and enjoying life. This will thrill them and will reframe your own reference point. It has also been said that parents are only ever as happy as is their least-happy child. Show them you are flourishing in your life. Remember the sacrifices they made for you.

- If you are in a committed relationship, honor the caretaker role your significant other undoubtedly selflessly fulfills. Find a day now and then where you do everything for him or her. Make the meals and clean the house. Do the chores he or she hates the most, be they washing windows, changing the beds, or mowing the lawn. If you don't know what those chores are, find out. Put on their favorite music. Watch their favorite movies with them (you make the popcorn and open up the wine). Take them for a Sunday drive. Surprise them with a small thank-you gift. Make them hot cocoa on a cold winter's night. You get the idea!

CHAPTER FORTY

You Had Me
at Hello

Stifled Romance and Intimacy

"Come gentle night,
come, loving, black-browed night,
Give me my Romeo;
and when he shall die, take him and cut him into little stars,
And he will make the face of heaven so fine
That all the world will be in love with night,
And pay no worship to the garish sun."

—*William Shakespeare,* Romeo and Juliet

Young men and women are primed for romance and connection. They are attractive, healthy and energized, and in the prime of their reproductive years. The mid-twenties to the late thirties is the stuff of every romance novel and "romcom" movie. At this age, sexual drive can be incandescent and irresistible. It is an absolute biological imperative. Whole industries revolve around accentuating or promoting the attractiveness of the age (clothing, lingerie, makeup, perfumes and colognes, music, movies, gyms, etc.).

Intertwined within the physical desire is a powerful drive to connect emotionally and romantically. This is a time when young men and women fall in and out of love, and often eventually find that special "one." Every weekend you will find them in restaurants and nightclubs, engaged in mile-a-minute conversations and gazing into each other's eyes. Those who have left this golden stage of life often think back with such bittersweet wistfulness.

In contrast, life in medicine may feel like being condemned to a jail cell. As if sentenced for a crime, you exist in a world of sleeplessness, physical exhaustion, mental fatigue, stress, sickness, death, sorrow, bad food, bad smells, constant demand, unisex clothing, and lack of fresh air—surrounded by the antithesis of society's prevailing young, healthy, and romantic aesthetic: the elderly. At a time when your generational cohort is out almost nightly seeking romantic connection with each other, you are either on call, recovering from call, thinking about your next night on call, staying late to chart in the EMR, charting remotely in the EMR, or thinking about charting in the EMR. You are tired, distressed, and contemplating the unfinished workload that is constantly on your plate.

Due to your lack of time and energy, you may also have "let yourself go." You look down and see no washboard stomach—heck, you haven't been to a gym in five years. You can't fit into your jeans from college anymore. Your skin is pasty, dry, and sallow—your eyes, sunken and bordered by dark circles. You have not bought a fun and confidence-boosting new article of clothing since you were in early medical school. Your perfume is the foam handwash you slather on as you leave the last patient's room.

And here lies the rub. It is nearly impossible to have a "normal" young adult sex life as a physician. Likewise, the experiences of burgeoning emotional intimacy and romantic attraction are challenged and often warped. Like all things in medicine, the world of physical intimacy and nascent romance is fraught with hurriedness, lack of access, lack of focus, lack of concentration, lack of energy—as well as misreads, missed-cues, alienation, disappointments, and dispirited performances.

Meaningful physical intimacy, and certainly emotional connection, takes time and presence. It takes attention to someone other than oneself. One of the greatest aphrodisiacs of all is the notion that someone truly "gets" you and likes what they see. But residents and physicians are often too tired to "get" anyone. You sit across from your date on the rare night out and fret about work. The first glass of wine acts more like a tranquilizer dart than an aphrodisiac. In a situation where you are supposed to be keying in on all sorts of subtle verbal and non-verbal sensual and romantic cues, you are fighting to keep your eyes open.

What's more, you are prone to engaging in distorted physical and emotional intimacy, spurred by the lack of time and self-reflection. Hospitals often become little soap operas, filled with rushed physical interludes and oft-disastrous pseudo-romances. You are exhausted, out of shape, emotionally needy, and someone catches your eye across the ICU. He or she is actually signaling that they are attracted to you—even in your bedraggled state. The excitement of a possible connection wakes you up a bit and flatters you.

These encounters can be uniquely unsatisfying, yet they may also be addictive. Worse, you may interpret these liaisons as meaningful love. If you are unattached, you may become convinced that you have "found the one," only to find somewhere down the line (hopefully before any nuptials) that you are not in the slightest bit compatible. If you are already attached, you may throw away "the one" for this new thrill-ride; after all, your special someone at home doesn't get you, is fed up with your hours and fatigue, and is no longer interested in you physically—or so you tell yourself.

So far, we have focused on younger residents and physicians, but the problems described are not at all dissimilar for you if you are middle aged or older. What is more, during these years, the relationship at home may be under significant duress. You now have had a decade or two to run parallel lives with your partner. After all, your partner has had to develop his or her own interests and activities—mostly devoid of your company.

You may want to make up for the youthful experiences in intimacy that you missed out on so many years back, only to find that your partner has developed his or her own solar system of serious and yet rewarding engagement. And horror of horrors, you are no longer at the epicenter. You now want to play; your significant other wants to grow. Emotional and physical intimacy is hopelessly in a rut. You become convinced that your partner is no longer attracted to you, and the fact that you are not intimately connecting only acts as confirming data. Someone young, exciting, and enticing catches your eye, and troubles begin.

Here are a few questions for you to contemplate and discuss with your peers, friends, families, mentors, or perhaps a therapist. Please see www.studergroup.com/thriving-physician for more questions.

Consider and Discuss

- What is the most romantic activity you can think of? What is the most sensual activity? When was the last time you engaged in these? List the ten most doable (on your budget) romantic activities. The ten most romantic nearby locations. The ten most sensual activities.

- If you look back at a night on the couch watching TV—how would it compare with a night of romance, passion, and physical intimacy?

- If you are living parallel lives with a partner, how can you merge the two? How can you pay honest, respectful, and meaningful homage to your partner's interests and schedule? How can you make sure your souls are still intertwining?

Building Resilience

We urge you to get with the game here! This is your time! No matter your age, you will never be this young and beautiful and slim and energized and fun-loving and vivacious again! If you give in to fatigue and inertia, you will miss out, and you will forever look back longingly and ruefully at what has been lost. No, you won't have the opportunities that many of your friends have to mingle and party and date. And you will disappoint some with your irregular and long hours. But this brilliant and electrifying world of physical and emotional attraction is just too special to miss. It is a most precious component of life, of experiencing the life force. It is truly lightning in a bottle.

So, when you get home on a Friday night tired, slimy, reeking, and already dreading a Saturday of call, shake it off. Get in the shower, soap up, rinse with cold water, and take in a big gulp of air. Get dressed and get out there!

- If you are single, join up with friends, go to a party, dance. Meet, flirt, and dance some more. Savor the thrill of the chase even if it leads nowhere.
- If you are attached, do the same, but with your partner! Revel in being alive and healthy. The work will still be there tomorrow. The patients will still be there tomorrow. Call will still be there tomorrow. At least you can deal with it with a smile on your face.
- If you are single, realize that in a medical center, there are a lot of young, single, attractive, and nice people. They may not look or act like it, all decked out in their hospital garb and all buried in their work, but many are looking for a real connection too. They are just

accustomed to your blitzing in and out of their workspace without so much as a "Hello, how are you today?"

- Slow down a bit, open your eyes, and exercise your vocal cords. Spend a few moments chatting. Offer a kind word or compliment now and then (please don't make it licentious or lascivious though!). Say something self-deprecating and funny now and then. Let people see what a friendly, sweet, witty bon vivant you really are.

- Casual hook-ups may be thrilling, but they are often the "lite" beer of intimacy. They can leave you feeling empty almost immediately afterwards and simply looking for more. Consider getting to know some of your coworkers a little before you get intimate. This may save you from some truly uncomfortable or even scary situations.

- If you are in a relationship, forget spontaneity. If you wait for a spark to ignite your passions, you will spend many an evening binging on Netflix and falling asleep by nine. Create a romance schedule and hold to it.

- Establish definitive *date nights* and make them real dates. Follow the wash-and-rinse instructions above. You too should dress to the nines. Change your look a bit for some variety. Be over-the-top romantic. Buy some flowers or a token gift. Employ some candlelight and wine. Experiment with new and exotic foods. Take a walk hand-in-hand on a beach (if you have one handy). Find an activity where you are both novices (e.g., pitch-and-putt golf) and laugh your way through it. Touch a lot, hug a lot, smooch a lot.

- Ask your significant other not to let you off the hook. Date nights are date nights, period. Even regular nights should involve some gestures of romance and intimacy. And you should be expected to turn off the TV and engage when your significant other asks you to.

- Keep a small journal of the romantic and/or sensual encounters you have over a three-month period (and no, you don't have to make it exceptionally detailed or name any names). After three months, review your journal. Ask yourself whether romance is a large part of your life, a small part, a rarely visited island, or a make-believe land you never experience.

CONCLUSION

Thriving in Your Medical Career

Concerns about physician suffering are resounding like cannon shots across all of medicine. Every hospital we visit, and every professional association we work with, is devoting increasing resources to trying to solve this problem. As we have noted, many creative efforts to improve efficiencies and ease practice burdens are being implemented. But the single most important determinant of your resilience, wellness, and happiness will be your own approach to, and interface with, your individual career environment. (And since there is no dividing line between the "professional you" and the "personal you," this also applies to your life outside of work.)

Our message throughout this book has been that you can indeed flourish throughout your career. The host of challenges and stressors you face daily in your medical career are protean and may seem rather daunting and oppressive at times. And yet, there is so much opportunity to thrive despite—and, at times, because of—these challenges that come with the life you have chosen. This is the core principle of personal resilience: the ability to come through stressful situations and times in as good a shape as you went in, *or better*! With each challenge discussed in the book, we have offered some hints as to how you might grow from encountering and engaging with them. Hopefully, some common themes have become apparent.

Learning to take care of yourself is central to the development of resilience. The importance of this cannot be overemphasized. Self-care does not come naturally, especially for physicians. You are scripted to care for others and to practice constant self-denial and delayed gratification. Breaking this resilience-draining cycle will take thoughtful effort for a long time.

Therefore, make it a routine to take inventory of your emotions, energy, and relationships—both at home and at work—and tend to them if they are lagging. When possible, take a break. Breathe in some fresh air, read a novel, go for a walk, take an extended weekend, meditate, exercise, paint, soak in a bath, go to a movie, play an instrument, call a friend—whatever it takes and for however long is needed to replenish your tanks of happiness, zeal, empathy, caring, and self-worth. And don't forget to care for the physical you. Remember to eat well, drink plenty of fluids, exercise some, and get enough sleep on a daily basis.

Also, maintain and expand your personal relationships. Gathering positive energy from your relationships at home and at work will fuel you through the toughest of times. Remember that as your relationships go, so will go your resilience. So, strengthen your bonds with loved ones. Do not allow the relationships that are important to you to slip away. Make time, manipulate your schedule, and extend yourself in order to spend meaningful moments with those you care about. Expand your circle of loved ones, build new friendships, repair damaged ones. At work, become an ambassador of collaboration and collegiality.

Building self and relationship resilience requires lifetime learning in two arenas: emotional intelligence and positive psychology. Knowing yourself and accepting the endless challenges to self-regulation (of your stress, communication, compulsions, and more) will be key to positively connecting with others both in and out of the workspace. This requires a combination of self-compassion and empathy. Treat yourself with interest, kindness, and forgiveness (and maybe a little self-deprecating humor); seek to understand and empathize with the emotional set point and the lot of others. When your antennae are finely tuned to the state of those around you, a resonance develops and a joy of collaboration will soon follow.

Positive psychology involves evaluating, trying, and emulating techniques and strategies that work for others who thrive in their environments, and you when you are at your best in your own. One very hearty such method: seeking daily uplifts. The day may be full of challenges, but it is also replete with uplifts—events and phenomena that can make you feel better and restore your psychic energy.

Try to focus less on the stressors and more on the occurrences that help dissipate stress. A smile from a coworker, a beautiful view through a nearby window, a compliment, a good clinical result, a text from a loved one, a newly learned fact, a thank you, or a funny anecdote will all serve this purpose. Make it a point to notice such things and count them up at the end of the day. Uplifts will counteract the challenges and remind you what a wonderful life you have.

Speaking of uplifts, remind yourself with frequency what a grand profession you are in. A career in medicine should offer you an everlasting supply of professional uplifts. After all, your day-to-day existence revolves around the care of others—most of whom are extraordinarily grateful for what you do for them. You impact people's lives. Your work has palpable *meaning*. And meaning is an antidote for burnout. Savor this. Never allow yourself to forget it. Find inspiration in it.

We hope that we have stirred you to view your career and your life from the perspective of *wonderment*—seeing the familiar in unfamiliar ways. Take a moment now and then and ponder what exactly is going on around you. You are on an amazing journey, working in a field full of scientific and technological miracles. We peer into the human body with exquisite fidelity. We safely engage in procedures that could not have even been dreamed about 100 years ago. We manipulate the very basic building blocks of life to save lives. It is and should be awe-inspiring, but to us it is all in a day's work. Allow yourself to be filled with wonder. Be a kid again, thrilled with discovery and brimming with excitement for the world around you.

We hope we have inspired you to look back, with wonderment and pride, on your personal and professional trek; to look forward with joyful anticipation about what is to come; and, more than anything, to look with deep appreciation at your current stage in your journey. Remind yourself frequently of all that you have achieved and where you are headed. You have done so much, and you do so much for so many people. Stop and savor this notion. You should feel proud; you are a testament to intelligence, industry, perseverance, caring, and grit. And you have a sterling future. Look at your life six months, five years, ten years down the road and envision it with great optimism and positivity. Map out your future and then follow the path you have blazed.

As you readjust your approach to the challenges of your career and begin to really thrive, you will notice many others who are not so lucky. Throw them a lifeline by building a "resilience team." There is real strength in numbers. With all the meaning, wonder, uplifts, and camaraderie available to you, the workday can offer periods of real joy. There's joy in helping others, in being part of something larger than yourself, in your own accomplishments, in simple yet profound human contact, in your growth, and so much more. It is so easy to miss the forest for the trees, but the opportunity for sustained joy in your own human experience surrounds you. Sample it, experience it, revel in it. Call upon it when things are down. Be thankful for it.

When joy is not forthcoming, and the path to your positive future seems obscure, utilize the available resources about you. Hospital systems, and healthcare organizations and societies, are taking burnout and the psychological toll of work-related stress very seriously. They are aligning an array of resources to be available to you. Familiarize yourself with these resources. Check out the available literature, websites, wellness teams, and professional support that are being offered.

Utilize professional assistance sooner rather than later if you feel you are headed down the wrong path. Intervention may be far more efficacious if engaged early rather than late in the course. There is no shame in seeking help. It is, in fact, a remarkably positive sign of emotional intelligence, self-compassion, and commitment to your patients—and to your own positive future.

For most of us, medicine is more of a calling than a career. Nevertheless, the "land mines" that fill the profession take their toll and threaten to leave us depleted of joy and meaning. Our hope is that this book will serve as a talisman for you throughout your journey—a reminder that, with a bit of mindful self- and relationship care, you can truly thrive.

Acknowledgments

We would like to acknowledge and thank the following individuals for their wonderful support and contributions to our book:

To Dan Smith, MD, for your thoughtful review of our advance manuscript.

To Studer Group, for your work to make healthcare a better place for all.

To Rebecca Fallon, Mary Sotile, Cindy Simonds, and Darla Summers, for your help in editing our earliest version of a tome into a manuscript worthy of submission for publication.

And finally, a special thanks to our great editors, Jamie Stewart and Dottie DeHart. You made our message better and helped our intention for this book shine through on every page.

References

We Need A Survival Guide! How This Book Came to Be (and Where We Hope to Go From Here)

1. Scudder, Laurie and Tait D. Shanagelt. "Two Sides of the Physician Coin: Burnout and Well-being." *Medscape*, February 9, 2015. https://www.medscape.com/viewarticle/839439.

2. Shapiro, Shauna L., Daniel E. Shapiro, and Gary Schwartz. "Stress Management in Medical Education: A Review of the Literature." *Academic Medicine* 75, no. 7 (2000): 48-59. https://journals.lww.com/academicmedicine/Fulltext/2000/07000/Stress_Management_in_Medical_Education__A_Review.23.aspx.

3. DeChant, Paul and Diane W. Shannon. *Preventing Physician Burnout: Curing the Chaos and Returning Joy to the Practice of Medicine.* North Charleston: Simpler Healthcare, 2016.

4. Sinsky, Christine A., Rachel Willard-Grace, Andrew M. Schutzbank, Thomas A. Sinsky, David Margolius, and Thomas Bodenheimer. "In Search of Joy in Practice: A Report of 23 High-Functioning Primary Care Practices." *Annals of Family Medicine* 11, no. 3 (2011): 272-278. doi:10.1370/afm.1531.

5. Studer, Quint and George Ford. *Healing Physician Burnout.* Pensacola: Fire Starter Publishing, 2015.

6. Swensen, Stephen, Andrea Kabcenell, and Tait Shanafelt. *Journal of Healthcare Management* 61, no. 2 (2016): 105-127. https://journals.lww.com/jhmonline/Abstract/2016/03000/Physician_Organization_Collaboration_Reduces.8.aspx.

7. Maslach, Christina, Susan E. Jackson, and Michael P. Leiter. The Maslach Burnout Inventory. 3rd ed. Palo Alto: Consulting Psychologists Press, 1996.

8. Shanafelt, Tait D. and John H. Noseworthy. "Executive Leadership and Physician Well-being: Nine Organizational Strategies to Promote Engagement and Reduce Burnout." *Mayo Clinic Proceedings* 92, no. 1 (2017): 129-146. doi:10.1016/j.mayocp.2016.10.004.

9. Shanafelt, Tait, Joel Goh, and Christine Sinsky. "The Business Case for Investing in Physician Well-being." *JAMA Internal Medicine* 177, no. 12 (2017): 1826-1832. doi:10.1001/jamainternalmed.2017.4340.

Introduction: It's a Doctor's Life for Me!

1. Schneider, Suzanne, Karen Kingsolver, and Jullia Rosdahl. "Can Physician Self-care Enhance Patient-centered Healthcare? Qualitative Findings from a Physician Well-being Coaching Program." *Journal of Family Medicine* 2, no. 1 (2015): 372-379. doi:10.1016/j.explore.2014.08.007.

2. Reivich, Karen J., Martin E. Seligman, and Sharon McBride. "Master Resilience Training in the U.S. Army." *American Psychologist* 66, no. 1 (2011): 25-34. doi:10.1037/a0021897.

3. Cornum, Rhonda, Michael D. Matthews, and Martin E. Seligman. "Comprehensive Soldier Fitness: Building Resilience in a Challenging Institutional Context." *American Psychologist* 66, no. 1 (2011): 4-9. doi:10.1037/a0021420.

4. McAbee, Joseph H., Brian T. Ragel, Shirley McCartney, Morgan Jones, L. Madison Michael II, Michael DeCuypere, Joseph S. Cheng, Frederick A. Boop, and Paul Kilmo Jr. "Factors Associated with Career Satisfaction and Burnout Among US Neurosurgeons: Results of a Nationwide Survey." *Journal of Neurosurgery* 123, no. 1 (2015): 161-173. doi:10.3171/2014.12.JNS141348.

5. Shanafelt, Tait D., Sonja Boone, Litjen Tan, Lotte N. Dyrbye, Wayne Sotile, Daniel Satele, Colin P. West, Jeff Sloan, and Michael R. Oreskovich. "Burnout and Satisfaction With Work-Life Balance Among US Physicians Relative to the General US Population." *Archives of Internal Medicine* 172, no. 18 (2012): 1377-1385. doi:10.1001/archinternmed.2012.3199.

6. Shanafelt, Tait D., Charles M. Balch, Gerald Bechamps, Tom Russell, Lotte Dyrbye, Daniel Satele, Paul Collicott, Paul J. Novotny, Jeff Sloan, and Julie Freishlag. "Burnout and Medical Errors Among American Surgeons." *Annals of Surgery* 251, no. 6 (2010): 995-1000. doi:10.1097/SLA.0b013e3181bfdab3.

7. West, Colin P., Mashele M. Huschka, Paul J. Novotny, Jeff A. Sloan, Joseph C. Kolars, Thomas M. Habermann, and Tait D. Shanafelt. "Association of Perceived Medical Errors With Resident Distress and Empathy: A Prospective Longitudinal Study." *Journal of the American Medical Association* 296, no. 9 (2006): 1071-1078. doi:10.1001/jama.296.9.1071.

8. Maslach, Christina, Susan E. Jackson, and Michael P. Leiter. *The Maslach Burnout Inventory.* 3rd ed. Palo Alto: Consulting Psychologists Press, 1996.

9. Gill, James. "Burnout: A Growing Threat in Ministry." *Human Development* 1, no. 2 (1980): 21-25.

10. Kraft, Urich. "Burned Out." *Scientific American Mind* 17, no. 3 (2006): 28–33. doi:10.1038/scientificamericanmind0606-28.

11. Maslach, Christina, Susan E. Jackson, and Michael P. Leiter. The Maslach Burnout Inventory. 3rd ed. Palo Alto: Consulting Psychologists Press, 1996.

12. Fallon, Rebecca S., Wayne M. Sotile, and Mary O. Sotile. *From Burnout to Resilience.* Davidson, NC: Sotile Center for Resilience, 2015.

13. Neff, Kristin. "The 5 Myths of Self-Compassion: What Keeps Us from Being Kinder to Ourselves?" *Psychotherapy Networker*, September/October 2015, 31-36.

Chapter 1 – Spring Forward? Can't We *Fall* Back? Time Compression – Time Starvation

1. Shanafelt, Tait D., Omar Hasan, Lotte N. Dyrbye, Christine Sinsky, Daniel Satele, Jeff Sloan, and Colin P. West. *Mayo Clinic Proceedings* 90, no. 12 (2015): 1600–1613. doi:10.1016/j.mayocp.2015.08.023.

2. Saad, Lydia. "The '40-Hour' Workweek Is Actually Longer -- by Seven Hours." *Gallup Economy*, August 29, 2014. https://news.gallup.com/poll/175286/hour-workweek-actually-longer-seven-hours.aspx.

Chapter 2 – Another Assignment? Gee, Thanks! The Curse of Multi-Tasking

1. Rogers, Robert and Stephen Monsell. "The Costs of a Predictable Switch Between Simple Cognitive Tasks." *Journal of Experimental Psychology: General* 124, no. 2 (1995): 207-231. doi:10.1037/0096-3445.124.2.207.

2. Miller, Earl. "Here's Why You Shouldn't Multitask, According to an MIT Neuroscientist." *Fortune*, December 8, 2016. http://fortune.com/2016/12/07/why-you-shouldnt-multitask.

Chapter 4 – You Want Me to Come See What? The Tyranny of Call

1. Shanafelt, Tait D., Sonja Boone, Litjen Tan, Lotte N. Dyrbye, Wayne Sotile, Daniel Satele, Colin P. West, Jeff Sloan, and Michael R. Oreskovich. "Burnout and Satisfaction with Work-Life Balance Among US Physicians Relative to the General US Population." *Archives of Internal Medicine* 172, no. 18 (2012): 1377-1385. doi:10.1001/archinternmed.2012.3199.

2. Dyrbye, Liselotte N., Prathibha Varkey, Sonja L. Boone, Daniel V. Satele, Jeff A. Sloan, and Tait D. Shanafelt. "Physician Satisfaction and Burnout at Different Career Stages." *Mayo Clinic Proceedings* 88, no. 12 (2013): 1358-1367. doi:10.1016/j.mayocp.2013.07.016.

Chapter 6 – ZZZZ: Sleep Deprivation and Sleep Deficit

1. Baldwin, Dewitt C. and Steven R. Daugherty. "Sleep Deprivation and Fatigue in Residency Training: Results of a National Survey of First- And Second-Year Residents." *Sleep* 27, no. 2 (2004): 217-223.

2. Philibert, Ingrid. "Sleep Loss and Performance in Residents and Non-Physicians: A Meta-Analytic Examination." *Sleep* 28, no. 11 (2005): 1392-1402.

3. Baldwin, Dewitt C. and Steven R. Daugherty. "Sleep Deprivation and Fatigue in Residency Training: Results of a National Survey of First- And Second-Year Residents." *Sleep* 27, no. 2 (2004): 217-223.

4. Sargent, M. Catherine, Wayne M. Sotile, Mary O. Sotile, Harry Rubash, Peter S. Vezeridis, Larry Harmon, and Robert L. Barrack. "Managing Stress in the Orthopaedic Family: Avoiding Burnout, Achieving Resilience." *Journal of Bone and Joint Surgery* 93, no. 8 (2011): 40. doi:10.2106/jbjs.j.01252.

5. Sargent, M. Catherine, Wayne M. Sotile, Mary O. Sotile, Harry Rubash, and Robert L. Barrack. "Stress and Coping Among Orthopaedic Surgery Residents and Faculty." *Journal of Bone and Joint Surgery* 86, no. 7 (2004): 1579-1586. https://journals.lww.com/jbjsjournal/Abstract/2004/07000/stress_and_coping_among_orthopaedic_surgery.32.aspx.

6. Dawson, Drew and Kathryn Reid. "Fatigue, Alcohol and Performance Impairment." *Nature* 388 (1997): 235-237. doi: 10.1038/40775.

7. Taffinder, Nick J., Ian Christopher McManus, Yilmaz Gul, Ronald Christopher Gordon Russell, and Ara Darzi. "Effect of Sleep Deprivation on Surgeons' Dexterity on Laparoscopy Simulator." *Lancet* 352, no. 9135 (1998): 1191. doi:10.1016/S0140-6736(98)00034-8.

8. Kozer, Eran, Dennis Scolnik, Alison Macpherson, Tara Keays, Kevin Shi, Tracy Luk, and Gideon Koren. "Variables Associated with Medication Errors in Pediatric Emergency Medicine." *Pediatrics* 110, no. 4 (2002): 737-742. http://pediatrics.aappublications.org/content/110/4/737.

9. Lockley, Steven W., Laura K. Barger, Najib T. Ayas, Jeffrey M. Rothschild, Charles A. Czeisler, and Christopher P. Landrigan. "Effects of Health Care Provider Work Hours and Sleep Deprivation on Safety and Performance." *Joint Commission Journal on Quality and Patient Safety* 33, no. 11 (2007): 7-18. doi:10.1016/S1553-7250(07)33109-7.

10. Fryer, Bronwyn. "Sleep Deficit: The Performance Killer." *Harvard Business Review,* October 2006. https://hbr.org/2006/10/sleep-deficit-the-performance-killer.

11. Prather, Aric A., Denise Janicki-Deverts, Martica H. Hall, and Sheldon Cohen. "Behaviorally Assessed Sleep and Susceptibility to the Common Cold." *Sleep* 38, no. 9 (2015): 1353-1359. doi:10.5665/sleep.4968.

12. Cappuccio, Francesco P., Daniel Cooper, Lanfranco D'Elia, Pasquale Strazzullo, and Michelle A. Miller. "Sleep Duration Predicts Cardiovascular Outcomes: A Systematic Review and Meta-Analysis of Prospective Studies." *European Heart Journal* 32, no. 12 (2011): 1484-1492. doi:10.1093/eurheartj/ehr007.

13. Nelson, Douglas. "Prevention and Treatment of Sleep Deprivation Among Emergency Physicians." *Pediatric Emergency Care* 23, no. 7 (2007): 498-503. doi:10.1097/01.pec.0000280519.30570.fa.

14. Minors, David S. and Jim M. Waterhouse. "Anchor Sleep as a Synchronizer of Rhythms on Abnormal Routines." *International Journal of Chronobiology* 7, no. 3 (1981): 165-188.

15. Amin, Mohammad M., Mark Graber, Khalid Ahmad, Dragos Manta, Sayeed Hossain, Zuzana Belisova, William Cheney, Morris S. Gold, and Avram R. Gold. "The Effects of a Mid-Day Nap on the Neurocognitive Performance of First-Year Medical Residents: A Controlled Interventional Pilot Study." *Academic Medicine* 87, no. 10 (2012): 1428-1433. doi:10.1097/ACM.0b013e3182676b37.

16. "Sleep Hygiene." National Sleep Foundation. Accessed March 7, 2015. http://sleepfoundation.org/ask-the-expert/sleep-hygiene.

17. The Epworth Sleepiness Scale. "About the ESS." http://epworthsleepinessscale.com/about-the-ess.

Chapter 9 – Your Worst Nightmare: The Torment of Bad Outcomes

1. Institute of Medicine. *To Err is Human: Building a Safer Health System*. Washington, DC: The National Academies Press, 1999.

Chapter 10 – Hey Guys, Watch This! The Self-Denial/Overindulgence Cycle

1. Figley, Charles R., ed. *Compassion Fatigue: Coping with Secondary Traumatic Stress Disorder in Those Who Treat the Traumatized.* Brunner/Mazel Psychological Stress Series, no. 23. New York: Taylor & Francis Group, 1995.

Chapter 11 – Families Are the Compass That Guides Us: The Stress That Accompanies Starting and/or Maintaining Family Relations

1. Newport, Frank and Joy Wilke. "Desire for Children Still Norm in U.S." *Gallup Politics,* September 25, 2013. https://news.gallup.com/poll/164618/desire-children-norm.aspx.

2. Turner, Patricia L., Kimberly Lumpkins, Joel Gabre, Maggie J. Lin, Xinggang Liu, and Michael Terrin. "Pregnancy Among Women Surgeons: Trends Over Time." *Archives of Surgery* 147, no. 5 (2012): 474-479. doi:10.1001/archsurg.2011.1693.

3. Association of American Medical Colleges. 2017. "More Women Than Men Enrolled in U.S. Medical Schools in 2017." https://news.aamc.org/press-releases/article/applicant-enrollment-2017.

Chapter 12 – 50.7 Percent: Women in Medicine

1. Association of American Medical Colleges. 2017. "More Women Than Men Enrolled in U.S. Medical Schools in 2017." https://news.aamc.org/press-releases/article/applicant-enrollment-2017.

2. Carr, Phyllis L., Arlene S. Ash, Robert H. Friedman, Laura Szalacha, Rosalind C. Barnett, Anita Palepu, and Mark M. Moskowitz. "Faculty Perceptions of Gender Discrimination and Sexual Harassment in Academic Medicine." *Annals of Internal Medicine* 132, no. 11 (2000): 889-896. doi:10.7326/0003-4819-132-11-200006060-00007.

3. Gjerberg, Elisabeth and Lise Kjølsrød. "The Doctor–Nurse Relationship: How Easy Is It to Be a Female Doctor Co-Operating with a Female Nurse?" *Social Science and Medicine* 52, no. 2 (2001): 189-202. doi:10.1016/S0277-9536(00)00219-7.

4. Eloy, Jean Anderson, Peter F. Svider, Deepa V. Cherla, Lucia Diaz, Olga Kovalerchik, Kevin M. Mauro, Soly Baredes, and Sujana S. Chandrasekhar. "Gender Disparities in Research Productivity Among 9952 Academic Physicians." *Laryngoscope* 123, no. 8 (2013): 1865-1875. doi:10.1002/lary.24039.

Chapter 14 – Garbage In, Garbage Out: Information Overload

1. Tamir, Diana I., Emma M. Templeton, Adrian F. Ward, and Jamil Zaki. "Media Usage Diminishes Memory for Experiences." *Journal of Experimental Social Psychology* 76 (2018): 161-168. doi:10.1016/j.jesp.2018.01.006.

Chapter 15 – On a Runaway Train: Lack of Control

1. Kuper, Hannah and Michale Marmot. "Job Strain, Job Demands, Decision Latitude, and Risk of Coronary Heart Disease within the Whitehall II Study." *Journal of Epidemiology & Community Health* 57, no. 2 (2003): 147-153. doi:10.1136/jech.57.2.147.

2. Judkins, Sharon K. and Melba Ingram. "Decreasing Stress Among Nurse Managers: A Long-Term Solution." *Journal of Continuing Education in Nursing* 33, no. 6 (2002): 259-264. doi:10.3928/0022-0124-20021101-06.

Chapter 19 – Cowabunga, Dude: The Shock of Lost Youth

1. Polivy, Janet and C. Peter Herman. "If at First You Don't Succeed: Fales Hopes of Self-Change." *American Psychologist* 57, no. 9 (2002): 677-689. doi:10.1037/0003-066X.57.9.677.

Chapter 21 – Like Entering a Den of Vipers: Malpractice Litigation

1. Ciofu, Carmen. "The Frequency and Severity of Medical Malpractice Claims: High Risk and Low Risk Specialties." *Maedica* 6, no. 3 (2011): 230-231.

2. Charles, Sara C. and Eugene Kennedy. *Defendant: A Psychiatrist on Trial for Medical Malpractice.* New York: The Free Press, 1985.

Chapter 22 – When We Are the Problem: Abusive Physician Behavior (and the Abused Child Syndrome)

1. Glasser, Mark, Israel Kolvin, Douglas C. Campbell, Adrian Glasser, Ian Leitch and Simone E. Farrelly. "Cycle of Child Sexual Abuse: Links Between Being a Victim and Becoming a Perpetrator." *British Journal of Psychiatry* 179, no. 6 (2001): 482-494. doi:10.1192/bjp.179.6.482.

Chapter 26 – Living in a Digital World: The Supremacy of the Electronic Medical Record

1.   Robertson, Sandy L., Mark D. Robinson, and Alfred Reid. "Electronic Health Record Effects on Work-Life Balance and Burnout Within the I³ Population." *Journal of Graduate Medical Education* 9, no. 4 (2017): 479-484. doi:10.4300/JGME-D-16-00123.1.

Chapter 32 – Where Is the Love? On-the-Job Isolation and Loneliness

1.   Hawkley, Louise C. and John T. Cacioppo. "Loneliness Matters: A Theoretical and Empirical Review of Consequences and Mechanisms." *Annals of Behavioral Medicine* 40, no. 2 (2010): 218-227. doi:10.1007/s12160-010-9210-8.

2.   Cacioppo, John T., Louise C. Hawkley, L. Elizabeth Crawford, John M. Ernst, Mary H. Burleson, Ray B. Kowalewski, William B. Malarkey, Eve Van Cauter, and Gary G. Berntson. "Loneliness and Health: Potential Mechanisms." *Psychosomatic Medicine* 64, no. 3 (2002): 407-417.

Chapter 34 – You First! The Impact of Fear

1.   Bourne, Tom, Laure Wynants, Mike Peters, Chantal Van Audenhove, Dirk Timmerman, Ben Van Calster, and Maria Jalmbrant. "The Impact of Complaints Procedures on the Welfare, Health and Clinical Practise of 7926 Doctors in the UK: A Cross-Sectional Survey." *BMJ Open* 5, no. 1 (2015). doi: 10.1136/bmjopen-2014-006687.

Chapter 35 – I Believe, I Believe; It's Silly, But I Believe

1.   Greenfield, Emily A., George E. Vaillant, and Nadine F. Marks. "Do Formal Religious Participation and Spiritual Perceptions Have Independent Linkages with Diverse Dimensions of Psychological Well-Being?" *Journal of Health and Social Behavior* 50, no. 2 (2009): 196-212. doi:10.1177/002214650905000206.

2.   Cornum, Rhonda, Michael D. Matthews, and Martin E. Seligman. "Comprehensive Soldier Fitness: Building Resilience in a Challenging Institutional Context." *American Psychologist* 66, no. 1 (2011): 4-9. doi: 10.1037/a0021420.

Chapter 37 – Everybody's Got a Little Larceny Operating in Them: Ethical Challenges in "Everyday" Medicine

1.   Beauchamp, Tom L. and James F. Childress. *Principles of Biomedical Ethics*. 7th ed. New York: Oxford University Press, 2012.

Chapter 38 – Winning Isn't Everything; It's the Only Thing!: Perpetual Peak Performance

1. Sarker, Md. Moniruzzaman, Mohammad Sahabuddin, and Nafisa Kasem. "Non-Financial Factor of Measuring Organizational Performance Brings Long Term Financial Capability: An Experience from Bangladesh." *International Journal of Research in Commerce and Management* 3, no. 5 (2012): (39-41).

2. Lesyk, Jack L. *Developing Sport Psychology Within Your Clinical Practice: A Practical Guide for Mental Health Professionals*. San Francisco: Jossey-Bass, 1998.

Chapter 39 – My Work Is My Best Friend: The Decay of Close Relationships

1. Shanafelt, Tait D., Omar Hasan, Lotte N. Dyrbye, Christine Sinsky, Daniel Satele, Jeff Sloan, and Colin P. West. *Mayo Clinic Proceedings* 90, no. 12 (2015): 1600–1613. doi:10.1016/j.mayocp.2015.08.023.

2. Orlando, Julia Sotile, Wayne M. Sotile, and Mary O. Sotile. "The Physician Family Life Survey." *Physician Family*, Winter 2016.

Assistance with Building Your Resiliency Program

Dr. Sotile and Dr. Simonds have amassed a fascinating series of observations, investigational data, and anecdotes from their work across many organizations as well as with the Carilion Clinic-Virginia Tech Carilion Neurosurgery team, providers from other programs, visiting medical students, and undergraduates. They are delighted to share their experience through small or large group talks, seminars, and/or discussions.

To arrange such a session please contact:

Wayne M. Sotile, PhD	**Gary R. Simonds, MD, MHCDS**
The Center for Physician Resilience	Chief of Neurosurgery
P.O. Box 2290	Carilion Clinic-Virginia Tech Carilion
Davidson, NC 28036	School of Medicine
Office: 336-794-0230	Phone: 540-529-4276
Mobile: 336-462-3943	Email: grsimonds57@gmail.com
www.sotile.com	Email: garyrsimonds@gmail.com
Email: sotile@sotilemail.com	

Additional Resources

About Huron:

Huron is a global consultancy that helps our clients drive growth, enhance performance, and sustain leadership in the markets they serve. We partner with them to develop strategies and implement solutions that enable the transformative change our clients need to own their future.

Learn more at www.huronconsultinggroup.com.

About Studer Group, a Huron solution:

A recipient of the 2010 Malcolm Baldrige National Quality Award, Studer Group is an outcomes-based healthcare performance improvement firm that partners with healthcare organizations in the United States, Canada, and beyond, teaching them how to achieve, sustain, and accelerate exceptional clinical, operational, and financial results.

Working with Huron, we help to get the foundation right so organizations can build a sustainable culture that promotes accountability, fosters innovation, and consistently delivers a great patient experience and the best quality outcomes over time.

To learn more about Studer Group, visit www.studergroup.com or call 850-439-5839.

Coaching:

Studer Group coaches work with healthcare leaders to create an aligned culture accountable to achieving outcomes together. Working side-by-side, we help to establish, accelerate, and hardwire the necessary changes to create a culture of excellence. This leads to better transparency, higher accountability, and the ability to target and execute specific, objective results that organizations want to achieve.

Studer Group offers coaching based on organizational needs: Evidence-Based Leadership^{SM}, Health System, Emergency Department, Medical Group, and Rural Healthcare.

Learn more about Studer Group coaching by visiting www.studergroup.com/coaching.

Conferences:

Huron and Studer Group offer interactive learning events throughout the year that provide a fresh perspective from industry-leading keynote speakers and focused sessions that share evidence-based methods to improve consistency, reduce variance, increase engagement, and create highly profitable organizations. They also provide networking opportunities with colleagues and experts and help participants learn new competencies needed to continuously improve the quality and experience of patient-centered care.

Most learning events offer continuing education credits. Find out more about upcoming conferences and register at www.studergroup.com/conferences.

Speaking:

From large association events to exclusive executive training, Studer Group speakers deliver the perfect balance of inspiration and education for every audience. As experienced clinicians and administrators, each speaker has a unique journey to share filled with expertise on a variety of healthcare topics. This personal touch, along with hard-hitting healthcare improvement tactics, empowers your team to take action.

Learn more about Studer Group speakers by visiting www.studergroup.com/speaking.

Publishing:

Studer Group offers practical, purpose-driven books that help healthcare professionals develop the skills they need to improve and sustain results across their organizations. For over 15 years, our resources have addressed industry challenges, elevated care delivery, and provided solutions for quality patient experiences.

With more than two million publications in circulation across the United States, Canada, Australia, New Zealand, China, and Japan, we are a trusted source for proven tactics and tools to help improve employee engagement, build leadership skills, and improve channels of communication.

Explore our catalog of resources by visiting www.publishing.studergroup.com.

Additional Offerings:

Healthcare leaders are facing unprecedented pressures that require changing care initiatives, payment models, and caregiver evaluations. Balancing these challenges as leaders address patient expectations of improved and on-demand access to quality care at a better price can seem daunting. That's why Studer Group created innovative solutions to help organizations anticipate and manage these pressures, so leaders can successfully own their future rather than being disrupted by it. From CXO Development Institutes to Care Transition Intensives to High-Reliability Programs to Perioperative Services to Post-Acute Offerings, Studer Group experts will work side-by-side to plan and execute.

View all of our offerings at www.studergroup.com.

About the Authors

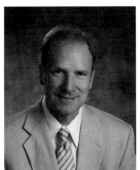

Gary R. Simonds, MD, MHCDS, is a highly experienced clinical and academic neurosurgeon. He trained at Walter Reed National Military Medical Center and completed a medical research fellowship at the Walter Reed Army Institute of Research. He also holds a master's degree in health care delivery science from Dartmouth College.

Dr. Simonds has practiced at Walter Reed and at the Geisinger Clinic. He is currently chief of neurosurgery at Carilion Clinic-Virginia Tech Carilion School of Medicine. He originally developed, and has run for the past 10 years, the Virginia Tech Carilion Neurosurgery Residency Training Program. He is a professor at the Virginia Tech Carilion School of Medicine, the Virginia Tech School of Neuroscience, and the Edward Via College of Osteopathic Medicine.

Known for his compassion and broad neurosurgical expertise, Dr. Simonds has personally performed over 13,500 operations, adult and pediatric. His interests have included socioeconomic issues affecting patient care, medical ethics, education of all levels of learners, and the promotion of wellness in medical practitioners and trainees.

He is active in many national neurosurgical committees, courses, and societies, and routinely presents nationally on subjects ranging from brain tumor research to ethics in healthcare delivery to compassionate care to innovations in education to resilience-building in healthcare providers.

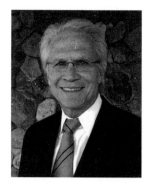

Wayne M. Sotile, PhD, is an international thought leader on physician resilience and one of the world's most seasoned clinicians specializing in life coaching for physicians and medical families. Over the past 35 years, he and his group have coached and counseled over 14,000 physicians. He is a pioneer in the field of clinical and health psychology.

A former faculty member of the Wake Forest School of Medicine, Dr. Sotile is the founder of the Sotile Center for Resilience and the Center for Physician Resilience in Davidson, North Carolina. He consults nationally with healthcare organizations and medical group practices concerned about resilience. He serves as a clinical assistant professor in the Department of Orthopaedic Surgery at Tulane University School of Medicine and as a special consultant in physician leadership and development for Atrium Health (formerly Carolinas HealthCare System) and FirstHealth of the Carolinas.

He has coauthored nine books, including *The Resilient Physician, The Medical Marriage,* and *Letting Go of What's Holding You Back,* and he is published widely in the peer-reviewed medical literature on topics related to physician burnout and medical family life.

Dr. Sotile has received lifetime career achievement awards from the American Academy of Medical Administrators and other healthcare professional societies. He has delivered more than 8,000 invited addresses to medical organizations throughout the country. Since 2007, Dr. Sotile has also served as a featured Studer Group speaker.